Updates in Clinical Dermatology

Series Editors

John Berth-Jones
Chee Leok Goh
Howard I. Maibach

More information about this series at http://www.springer.com/series/13203

Steven R. Feldman • Abigail Cline
Adrian Pona • Sree S. Kolli

Editors

Treatment Adherence in Dermatology

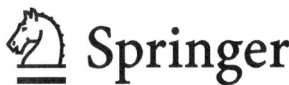 Springer

Editors
Steven R. Feldman, MD, PhD
Departments of Dermatology, Pathology and Social
Sciences & Health Policy
Wake Forest School of Medicine
Winston-Salem, NC
USA

Adrian Pona, MD
Department of Dermatology
Wake Forest School of Medicine
Winston-Salem, NC
USA

Abigail Cline, MD, PhD
Department of Dermatology
Wake Forest School of Medicine
Winston-Salem, NC
USA

Sree S. Kolli, BA
Department of Dermatology
Wake Forest School of Medicine
Winston-Salem, NC
USA

ISSN 2523-8884   ISSN 2523-8892   (electronic)
Updates in Clinical Dermatology
ISBN 978-3-030-27808-3   ISBN 978-3-030-27809-0   (eBook)
https://doi.org/10.1007/978-3-030-27809-0

This Springer imprint is published by the registered company Springer Nature Switzerland AG
The registered company address is: Gewerbestrasse 11, 6330 Cham, Switzerland

Preface

Successful medical care rests upon three pillars: making the right diagnosis, prescribing the right treatment, and getting patients to take the medication. Medical school and postgraduate training focus heavily on two of those elements: making the right diagnosis and prescribing the right medication. Far less attention—much too little—is paid to what it takes to get patients to take their medication.

As a result, the foundation for treatment success is rotten, and too often patients have less than optimal outcome because they have less than optimal adherence to treatment. Everyone knows this—including patients, doctors, pharmaceutical companies, insurers, and government regulators. Everyone wants adherence to be better. Improving adherence would be a win-win-win for all concerned.

How can we get there? Thích Nhất Hạnh, a Vietnamese Buddhist, had some very good advice: "When you plant lettuce, if it does not grow well, you don't blame the lettuce. You look for reasons it is not doing well. It may need fertilizer or more water or less sun. You never blame the lettuce." Blaming the patient for poor adherence is not helpful. The responsibility is on us. The way we in the healthcare system prescribe medication is simply not a good approach for getting patients to take their treatment.

In this book, we discuss how poor adherence to treatment is or, in other words, how poorly we in the healthcare system are at getting our patients to take medication. We describe novel, basic, fundamental truths about what must be done to have any hope of getting patients to take medication well. We focus on practical tools and advance psychological methods to help patients achieve what we all want: better adherence and better outcomes.

Winston Salem, NC, USA

Steven R. Feldman
Abigail Cline
Adrian Pona
Sree S. Kolli

Acknowledgments

We would like to thank Raj Balkrishnan, Scott Davis, Christie Carroll, Leah Cardwell, Elias Oussedik, and the other fellows who have conducted adherence research at Wake Forest. We would also like to thank Dr. Joe Jorizzo, Dr. Alan Fleischer, and Dr. Amy McMichael for their ongoing support, mentorship, and contribution to our research. Lastly, we would like to thank all of the students who have helped us with our research.

Contents

Contributors

Abigail Cline, MD, PhD Department of Dermatology, Wake Forest School of Medicine, Winston-Salem, NC, USA

Steven R. Feldman, MD, PhD Departments of Dermatology, Pathology and Social Sciences & Health Policy, Wake Forest School of Medicine, Winston-Salem, NC, USA

Katelyn R. Glines, BS Center for Dermatology Research, Department of Dermatology, Wake Forest School of Medicine, Winston-Salem, NC, USA

Wasim Haidari, BS, BA Center for Dermatology Research, Department of Dermatology, Wake Forest School of Medicine, Winston-Salem, NC, USA

Spencer Hawkins, MD Department of Dermatology, University of Michigan, Ann Arbor, MI, USA

Sree S. Kolli, BA Department of Dermatology, Wake Forest School of Medicine, Winston-Salem, NC, USA

E. J. Masicampo, PhD Department of Psychology, Wake Forest University, Winston-Salem, NC, USA

Adrian Pona, MD Department of Dermatology, Wake Forest School of Medicine, Winston-Salem, NC, USA

Eugenie Y. Quan, BA Center for Dermatology Research, Department of Dermatology, Wake Forest School of Medicine, Winston-Salem, NC, USA

Vignesh Ramachandran, BS Center for Dermatology Research, Department of Dermatology, Wake Forest School of Medicine, Winston-Salem, NC, USA

Monica Shah, BSc Faculty of Medicine, University of Toronto, Toronto, ON, Canada

Lindsay C. Strowd, MD Center for Dermatology Research, Department of Dermatology, Wake Forest School of Medicine, Winston-Salem, NC, USA

Felicia Tai, BMSc Faculty of Medicine, University of Toronto, Toronto, ON, Canada

Bernard Vrijens, PhD AARDEX Group, The Labs, Liège Science Park, Liège, Belgium

Chapter 1
Reasons for Nonadherence

Adrian Pona, Abigail Cline, and Steven R. Feldman

Introduction

Poor patient adherence is especially challenging in the field of dermatology, where only 50% of patients with chronic skin conditions adhere to the treatment plan outlined by their provider [1]. About one-third of patients never redeem their prescriptions from a dermatology clinic. Even if patients do fill the prescriptions, adherence often drops off after a few days. Poor adherence leads to poor health outcomes and increased financial expenditure for patients. By recognizing and addressing common barriers to treatment adherence, providers may help patients successfully incorporate and adhere to treatment regimens. Improving patient adherence may provide a convenient way to improve patient outcomes and decrease healthcare costs.

While there are various reasons for nonadherence, one conceptual model of barriers to adherence focus on patient, prescriber, and healthcare system factors [2]. Nonadherence can also be categorized into three phases: *initiation*, *implementation*, and *persistence*. *Initiation* includes failure to fill and begin taking a prescription [3]. *Implementation* is the patient's ability to agree, comprehend, and translate the healthcare provider's instructions. Finally, *persistence* involves maintaining the recommended treatment regimen [3, 4].

This chapter will first discuss barriers specific to patients, providers, and healthcare systems, then it will discuss common barriers that are shared between patients and providers.

Patient-Centered Barriers

Patient barriers create a significant practice gap in all specialties. A patient-centered approach may help providers investigate potential risks for nonadherence. To bridge practice gaps, patient barriers must be recognized. Patients may fail to take their medication unintentionally or intentionally. Unintentional nonadherence may be related to forgetfulness, complex treatment regimens, and

A. Pona (✉) · A. Cline
Department of Dermatology, Wake Forest School of Medicine, Winston-Salem, NC, USA
e-mail: apona@wakehealth.edu

S. R. Feldman
Departments of Dermatology, Pathology and Social Sciences & Health Policy, Wake Forest School of Medicine, Winston-Salem, NC, USA

© Springer Nature Switzerland AG 2020
S. R. Feldman et al. (eds.), *Treatment Adherence in Dermatology*, Updates in Clinical Dermatology, https://doi.org/10.1007/978-3-030-27809-0_1

Table 1.1 Intentional and Unintentional Reasons for Nonadherence [1–14]

Intentional	Unintentional
Patient beliefs	Forgetfulness
Fear of adverse effects	Lack of health-related education
Patient preference	Psychiatric illnesses
Complex treatment regimen	Poor communication
Medication cost	Failure to refill medication
Insurance difficulties	Limited access to healthcare
Poor patient-physician relationship	Poor patient-physician relationship

psychiatric illnesses [5–8]. Reasons for intentional nonadherence may include patient beliefs, fear of adverse effects, and patient preference (Table 1.1) [9].

A patient's beliefs can influence whether they initiate, implement, and persist with therapy. A patient may believe he received the wrong diagnosis, and therefore wrong medication, from his provider. If a patient feels he was not adequately examined and understood, he may be less likely to fill or take the suggested medication. A patient might also believe his condition is only temporary, and therefore prematurely stop therapy after some improvement. This can be especially challenging in chronic conditions that require continuous treatments [10].

A common reason for intentional nonadherence is a patient's fear of adverse effects due to the medication [11]. "Steroid phobia" describes negative feelings and beliefs about using topical corticosteroids. Common concerns about topical corticosteroids include skin thinning, the potential of topical corticosteroids to affect growth and development, and nonspecific long-term effects [12]. In one study, prevalence of steroid phobia in caregivers of children with atopic dermatitis (AD) reached about 38% [12]. If patients or caregivers fear of the topical corticosteroid side effect profile, they may be less willingness to use the medication as prescribed.

Patient preferences can impact adherence; therefore, a patient-centered approach may be helpful. Addressing and reconciling patient goals and preferences can help providers and patients agree on a feasible treatment regimen [13]. For example, some patients with severe psoriasis may prefer oral over injectable medications, even if the injectable medication is more likely to result in better disease control. Patient preference of a particular vehicle formulation for their topical medication may also impact their level of adherence [14, 15]. Subjects satisfied with their prescribed medication are more adherent than unsatisfied subjects ($P < 0.001$) [16].

Prescriber-Centered Barriers

Although the responsibility for poor adherence is often placed on patients, there is much that physicians and the healthcare system can do to enhance adherence behavior (Table 1.2). Providers may contribute to patients' poor adherence by prescribing expensive medications that patients cannot afford, recommending complex regimens that are difficult to follow, and failing to adequately educate patients on the medication's benefits and side effects. All of these factors lead to a poor patient-provider relationship, which can also result in poor adherence [11]. By recognizing and addressing provider-specific barriers, providers can standardize how they prescribe and improve adherence outcomes in patients.

The high cost of prescription drugs means many patients cannot afford their medications. Patient may fail to pick up their medications, skip doses to make the medication last longer, or stop treatment early due to the cost. However, providers are often unaware how much medications will cost patients. Providers and patients often fail to seek out pricing information before filling prescriptions. Prescribing generic prescriptions increases the likelihood that the patient can afford a medication [17].

Table 1.2 Patient, prescriber, and Healthcare-Centered Barriers to adherence [1–9, 11–18]

Patient-centered barrier	Prescriber-centered barrier	Healthcare-centered barrier
Forgetfulness	Complex treatment regimen	Limited access to healthcare
Psychiatric illness	Prescribing high cost medications	Restricted formularies
Patient beliefs	Poor communication	Medication cost
Fear of adverse effects		Switching formularies
Patient preference		Copayments

Complex treatment regimens often confuse patients and decrease their motivation, leading to poor adherence. Prescribing multiple medications after one office visit or adding prescriptions on top of a large list of medications, can reduce patient adherence. Simplifying treatment regimens reduces the burden of treatment and increases the likelihood that patients will adhere. Patients are more likely to follow a once daily treatment compared to twice daily. Combination medications also reduces the burden of treatment and increases adherence [11, 18, 19].

Poor communication by the provider to the patient can also result in poor adherence. Providers may not adequately explain the patient's condition, the need for medication, treatment expectations, and potential adverse effects. Patient education is be a key component of the clinical encounter. It offers an opportunity to address patient concerns and build a strong patient-provider relationship. By failing to communicate basic information, healthcare providers may jeopardize a patient's disease and treatment understanding and overall adherence [11, 20, 21].

Prescribers who fail to create a strong bond with their patient may increase the risk of nonadherence. Using a patient-centered approach may strengthen trust between both parties and prevent a poor patient-provider relationship [11, 22–24].

Healthcare-Centered Barriers

Healthcare-associated barriers to adherence include limited access to healthcare, restricted formularies, switching to a different formulary, and high costs for medications, copayments, or both [25–27]. The patient, provider, pharmacies, hospitals, insurance, and pharmaceutical companies are all components of the healthcare system [28].

Factor that create poor access to healthcare— including living in an area with poor access, lack of transportation, lack of adequate insurance, financial issues, and absence of other resources— also influence adherence [17, 29]. Other healthcare-associated factors that may influence adherence include extensive waitlist for an appointment with a specialist, lengthy wait time within the clinic, and confusing healthcare referral systems [30–32].

Insurance also has a strong influence on healthcare-associated nonadherence. Insurance issues include difficulty finding in-network healthcare providers, drug plans that do not cover certain prescription medications, and unaffordable copayment [11, 22, 23, 33]. For example, providers may not prescribe the best medication if it does not fall in a patient's restricted network formulary [34]. Such limitations impact the patient, provider, and healthcare system.

Common Barriers of Patients and Providers

Most adherence barriers are described as patient-oriented, but reframing common barriers as provider-oriented can help physicians influence adherence [11]. The focus of this section is to identify and discuss barriers to medication adherence that are common to both patients and providers

Table 1.3 Common barriers for patients and providers [6]

Patient	Provider
Treatment education	
Poor health literacy	Poor communication skills
Beliefs and perception of symptoms	
Fear of adverse effects	Believing patients are adherent
Treatment dissatisfaction	Failure to acknowledge patient beliefs
Forgetfulness	
Failure to remember regimen	Failure to provide instructions
Psychiatric illness	
Depression	Failure to recognize psychiatric comorbidities
Anxiety	Failure to provide appropriate referrals
Cost and insurance	
Lack of insurance	Writing expensive prescriptions
Expensive copay	Failure to provide patient assistance
Complex treatment regimen	
Polypharmacy	Prescribing multiple medications
Inability to follow instructions	Failure to offer prompt return visit

(Table 1.3). Examining shared barriers from both patients and providers highlights each of their specific responsibilities to address these concerns.

Treatment Education

Patient

Poor patient education is a common cause of unintentional nonadherence [4]. Patients may have insufficient understanding of the reasons, benefits, and adverse effects of the prescription medication [17]. A patient's capacity to process and understand basic medical information is defined as health literacy. [35, 36] In the United States, an estimated 90 million have poor health literacy skills [37]. In a study investigating health literacy in the United States, 12% of adults had proficient health literacy, 53% had intermediate, 22% had basic, and 14% had below basic health literacy [38]. Limited health literacy is associated with poorer patient-physician communication, health-related skills, and health outcomes. Poor health literacy is also associated with nonadherence [39]. Patients may not understand the importance of continuously using their medication in chronic conditions, as the terms controlled and cured may be confusing [40]. When psoriasis subjects were asked about their reasons for not applying topical corticosteroids, 20% reported inadequate knowledge about their disease [16]. Recognizing poor health literacy and explaining the rationale behind the prescribed medication can bridge patient education gaps.

Provider

There is a link between patient adherence and provider-patient communication, Communication contributes to the patients' understanding of the illness, the need for medication, and the risks and benefits of treatment. However, if a provider insufficiently addresses these areas, patients may leave feeling confused about their diagnosis, their medication, and their treatment plan [17]. Providers may also cause nonadherence by not providing a definitive diagnosis, providing too much information, or avoiding simple language [4, 41, 42].

One study investigated whether dermatologists provide inadequate education to their patients. A checklist containing diagnosis, treatment duration, frequency of application, dosage, drug effect, medication name, and possible adverse effects assessed whether the physician provided basic education. Patients were then asked about their education 10 days after the clinic visit. During the clinic visit, no physician mentioned drug price or potential adverse effects, and only 18% of physicians mentioned dosage. While all physicians mentioned the medication name and frequency of application, only 65% mentioned diagnosis and treatment duration. At Day 10, 12% of subjects knew the medication dosage, 35% knew treatment duration, 41% knew their diagnosis, 47% were concerned about side effects, and 71% knew the application frequency [20].

Beliefs and Perception of Symptoms

Patient

Patient beliefs, such as misconception of disease severity, perceived ineffectiveness of treatment, and fear of adverse effects, can impede patient adherence [43, 44]. Some patients believe they are invulnerable to illness and therefore refuse the recommended treatment [45]. Other patients stop treatment prematurely because they believe the treatment is ineffective. Common reasons for nonadherence in psoriasis patients include perceived low efficacy of treatment, time consuming regimens, and poor aesthetic appearance of treatment [46]. Patient belief of disease clearance can cause patients to decrease their dosage or completely discontinue treatment [4]. If patients do not perceive therapeutic effectiveness from their treatment, their motivation and adherence, to treatment could decrease.

Provider

Healthcare provider's assumption that their patient is adherent may pose a barrier. A cross-sectional study explored how many primary care providers believed that their patients were adherent to their medication and how many of those patients were actually adherent. About 50% of primary care providers incorrectly estimated that their patients were adherent to their medication. Of the primary care providers who incorrectly estimated, providers were more likely to overestimate than underestimate the number of adherent patients ($P = 0.05$) [47]. Another study reported 9% of healthcare providers believed their patient would truthfully admit in failing to fill their prescription; however, 83% of patients admitted they do not mention their unfilled prescription to their primary care provider [48]. Reasons why patients might withhold such information include fear of embarrassment, punishment, or the provider's overreaction [40].

Forgetfulness

Patient

Forgetfulness may be the most common reason for nonadherence [49–53]. When acne subjects were asked why they were nonadherent, 66% specified "forgetting" their medication, and 15% stated they were just too busy [54]. In an online survey of psoriasis subjects being managed with biologic therapy, 44.4% of adalimumab treated subjects and 3.2% of ustekinumab treated subjects reported nonadherence secondary to forgetfulness [55]. Similar findings in AD reported 92% of subjects forgot to take their medication at one point in time [56].

Provider

Around 50% of patients cannot recall physician instructions after a clinical visit [57, 58]. Focusing patient management by improving forgetfulness through behavioral and commercial services may bridge this barrier to adherence [17]. Written action plans are a promising intervention to improve adherence. A prospective clinical trial enrolling 35 pediatric AD subjects were given an eczema action plan at baseline visit and were followed for 12 months. The action plan contained instructions on daily medication use. Efficacy was measured by disease severity. At 12 months, 80% of subjects improved and 68% of caregivers felt the action plan was helpful [59]. Commercial services that may help include reminder devices, mobile applications, games, and other modes of technology although efficacy is limited [60].

Psychiatric Illness

Patient

Depression may be a foremost predictor of adherence [11, 61]. Depression is more prevalent in psoriasis patients (9.1%) compared to the general population (5.4%, $P < 0.001$) [62]. Elderly patients with psoriasis suffering from depression are less likely to maintain adherence to topical corticosteroids ($P < 0.01$) [63]. In addition to depression, anxiety is prevalent in 6.3% of psoriasis subjects compared to non-psoriasis control ($P < 0.001$) [62]. Psoriasis patients with minimal anxiety have better adherence rates to biologic therapy than patients with severe anxiety [64]. Recognizing and acknowledging psychiatric comorbidities could improve treatment outcome.

Provider

Due to the prevalence of psychiatric comorbidities in dermatology, failure to recognize such limitations in the patient may jeopardize adherence and treatment outcome [62, 65–67]. Dermatologists do not routinely screen for depression, so the prevalence of depression in dermatology patients may be underestimated [68]. Recognizing depression in dermatology patients, recommending treatment of psychiatric illnesses, and referring them to proper mental health services during the clinical encounter may help improve quality of life and overall treatment outcome, as well as decrease the risk of non-adherence [17, 69].

Cost and Insurance

Patient

The most common reason for nonadherence in biologic therapy was cost. In survey responses, 18.5% of patients reported adalimumab as unaffordable, whereas 22.6% of patients reported ustekinumab as unaffordable [55]. Due to increasing drug costs, 11 to 26% of patients insured by Medicare skip doses, divide the medication dose, and refuse to fill the prescription [70–74]. Risk factors associated with financial-related nonadherence includes socioeconomic status, minorities, and comorbidities [72, 74, 75]. A cross-sectional survey study exploring cost-saving strategies that may influence adherence reported 39.6% of survey responders used at least one cost-saving strategy. Subjects who received free samples (OR = 1.18; P = 0.04), split their medication (OR = 1.45; P = 0.001), and were being managed with more than 10 medications (OR = 1.65; P < 0.0001) were more likely to be nonadherent [74]. Increased out-of-pocket spending increases the risk of nonadherence [76, 77].

Provider

The current nature of healthcare costs suggests a negative impact on drug prices, premiums, and poor drug coverage [78–80]. Such economic changes impact a patient's ability to adhere to their medication regimen as patients cannot take their prescribed medication when they cannot afford it. In only 2.2% of office visits do physicians ask how much a patient was paying for their medication, and in only about 1.4% of office visits do physicians ask patients if medication cost was a problem. Physicians provided a solution to the cost problem in about 17.9% of visits [81]. A similar study in an outpatient dermatology clinic stated no dermatologist mentioned drug costs while educating their patient [20]. Prescribing affordable generic medications and providing a number for the pharmacist to contact in case medications are too expensive are cost-saving approaches [17].

Complex Treatment Regimen

Patient

Complex treatment regimen may dissuade even the most motivated patient from adhering [11]. Polypharmacy, along with frequency, location of application, and dosage can complicate treatment outcome and adherence [4, 82, 83]. In dermatology, complex regimens may involve the use of multiple topical agents that need frequent application. Patients may become confused about which medications are for what location, and how often each medication should be applied. For example, although treatment of scalp psoriasis often involves multiple agents (e.g. topical corticosteroid, keratolytic agent), patient motivation to adhere may decrease with complicated instructions [84].

Provider

Poor provider awareness in prescribing complex treatment regimens may predispose to nonadherence. Although a tendency exists for physicians to add another medication when the initial treatment fails, having a short follow-up visit may offer providers an opportunity to discover the initial medication may have been too complex or burdensome for their patient. Such findings may help providers tailor their management appropriately [85]. Healthcare providers may influence adherence by offering fewer and simpler medications in shorter dosing schedules [17].

Conclusion

Intentional and unintentional reasons for nonadherence may be categorized into patient, prescriber, or healthcare-centered barriers. Providers may recognize and address such barriers to help prevent unfilled prescriptions, maintain treatment, and improve clinical outcome.

Conflicts of Interest Dr. Steven Feldman has received research, speaking and/or consulting support from a variety of companies including Galderma, GSK/Stiefel, Almirall, Leo Pharma, Boehringer Ingelheim, Mylan, Celgene, Pfizer, Valeant, Abbvie, Samsung, Janssen, Lilly, Menlo, Merck, Novartis, Regeneron, Sanofi, Novan, Qurient, National Biological Corporation, Caremark, Advance Medical, Sun Pharma, Suncare Research, Informa, UpToDate and National Psoriasis Foundation. He is founder and majority owner of www.DrScore.com and founder and part owner of Causa Research, a company dedicated to enhancing patients' adherence to treatment.

Dr. Adrian Pona and Dr. Abigail Cline have no conflicts to disclose.

References

1. Brown MT, Bussell JK. Medication adherence: WHO cares? Mayo Clin Proc. 2011;86(4):304–14.
2. Osterberg L, Blaschke T. Adherence to medication. N Engl J Med. 2005;353(5):487–97.
3. Vrijens B, De Geest S, Hughes DA, Przemyslaw K, Demonceau J, Ruppar T, et al. A new taxonomy for describing and defining adherence to medications. Br J Clin Pharmacol. 2012;73(5):691–705.
4. Feldman SR, Vrijens B, Gieler U, Piaserico S, Puig L, van de Kerkhof P. Treatment adherence intervention studies in dermatology and guidance on how to support adherence. Am J Clin Dermatol. 2017;18(2):253–71.
5. Nafradi L, Galimberti E, Nakamoto K, Schulz PJ. Intentional and unintentional medication non-adherence in hypertension: the role of health literacy, empowerment and medication beliefs. J Public Health Res. 2016;5(3):762.
6. Lehane E, McCarthy G. Intentional and unintentional medication non-adherence: a comprehensive framework for clinical research and practice? A discussion paper. Int J Nurs Stud. 2007;44(8):1468–77.
7. Sabate E. Adherence to long-term therapies. Evidence for action. Geneva: World Health Organization; 2003.
8. Horne R, Weinman J, Barber N, Elliot R, Morgan M. Adherence and compliance in medicine taking. Report for the National Coordinating Centre for NHS Service Delivery and Organization R and D (NCCSDO). 2005 [Available from: http://www.netscc.ac.uk/hsdr/files/project/SDO_FR_08-1412-076_V01.pdf.
9. Arts DL, Voncken AG, Medlock S, Abu-Hanna A, van Weert HC. Reasons for intentional guideline non-adherence: a systematic review. Int J Med Inform. 2016;89:55–62.
10. DiMatteo MR, Haskard KB, Williams SL. Health beliefs, disease severity, and patient adherence: a meta-analysis. Med Care. 2007;45(6):521–8.
11. Devine F, Edwards T, Feldman SR. Barriers to treatment: describing them from a different perspective. Patient Prefer Adherence. 2018;12:129–33.
12. Kojima R, Fujiwara T, Matsuda A, Narita M, Matsubara O, Nonoyama S, et al. Factors associated with steroid phobia in caregivers of children with atopic dermatitis. Pediatr Dermatol. 2013;30(1):29–35.
13. Wade R, Paton F, Woolacott N. Systematic review of patient preference and adherence to the correct use of graduated compression stockings to prevent deep vein thrombosis in surgical patients. J Adv Nurs. 2017;73(2):336–48.
14. Patel NU, D'Ambra V, Feldman SR. Increasing adherence with topical agents for atopic dermatitis. Am J Clin Dermatol. 2017;18(3):323–32.
15. Ellis RM, Koch LH, McGuire E, Williams JV. Potential barriers to adherence in pediatric dermatology. Pediatr Dermatol. 2011;28(3):242–4.
16. Gokdemir G, Ari S, Koslu A. Adherence to treatment in patients with psoriasis vulgaris: Turkish experience. J Eur Acad Dermatol Venereol. 2008;22(3):330–5.
17. Lewis DJ, Feldman SR. Practical ways to improve patient adherence. Columbia, SC: CreateSpace Independent Publishing Platform. 2017.
18. Shubber Z, Mills EJ, Nachega JB, Vreeman R, Freitas M, Bock P, et al. Patient-reported barriers to adherence to antiretroviral therapy: a systematic review and meta-analysis. PLoS Med. 2016;13(11):e1002183.
19. Vitalis D. Factors affecting antiretroviral therapy adherence among HIV-positive pregnant and postpartum women: an adapted systematic review. Int J STD AIDS. 2013;24(6):427–32.
20. Storm A, Benfeldt E, Andersen SE, Andersen J. Basic drug information given by physicians is deficient, and patients' knowledge low. J Dermatolog Treat. 2009;20(4):190–3.
21. Kardas P, Lewek P, Matyjaszczyk M. Determinants of patient adherence: a review of systematic reviews. Front Pharmacol. 2013;4:91.
22. Holtzman CW, Shea JA, Glanz K, Jacobs LM, Gross R, Hines J, et al. Mapping patient-identified barriers and facilitators to retention in HIV care and antiretroviral therapy adherence to Andersen's Behavioral Model. AIDS Care. 2015;27(7):817–28.
23. Brundisini F, Vanstone M, Hulan D, DeJean D, Giacomini M. Type 2 diabetes patients' and providers' differing perspectives on medication nonadherence: a qualitative meta-synthesis. BMC Health Serv Res. 2015;15:516.
24. O'Rourke G, O'Brien JJ. Identifying the barriers to antiepileptic drug adherence among adults with epilepsy. Seizure. 2017;45:160–8.

25. Meiners M, Tavares NUL, Guimaraes LSP, Bertoldi AD, Pizzol T, Luiza VL, et al. Access and adherence to medication among people with diabetes in Brazil: evidences from PNAUM. Rev Bras Epidemiol. 2017;20(3):445–59.
26. Shirneshan E, Kyrychenko P, Matlin OS, Avila JP, Brennan TA, Shrank WH. Impact of a transition to more restrictive drug formulary on therapy discontinuation and medication adherence. J Clin Pharm Ther. 2016;41(1):64–9.
27. Lee M, Salloum RG. Racial and ethnic disparities in cost-related medication non-adherence among cancer survivors. J Cancer Surviv. 2016;10(3):534–44.
28. Medication Adherence Tech: a dynamic and crowded market, but where are all the winners in the space? (Part 1 of 2) 2017. Available from: https://www.mobihealthnews.com/content/medication-adherence-tech-dynamic-and-crowded-market-where-are-winners-space-part-1-2.
29. Shafer PO, Buchhalter J. Patient education: identifying risks and self-management approaches for adherence and sudden unexpected death in epilepsy. Neurol Clin. 2016;34(2):443–56.. ix
30. McKenzie K, Forsyth K, O'Hare A, McClure I, Rutherford M, Murray A, et al. The relationship between waiting times and 'adherence' to the Scottish Intercollegiate Guidelines Network 98 guideline in autism spectrum disorder diagnostic services in Scotland. Autism. 2016;20(4):395–401.
31. Sears C, Andersson Z, Cann M. Referral systems to integrate health and economic strengthening services for people with HIV: a qualitative assessment in Malawi. Glob Health Sci Pract. 2016;4(4):610–25.
32. Kehler DS, Kent D, Beaulac J, Strachan L, Wangasekara N, Chapman S, et al. Examining patient outcome quality indicators based on wait time from referral to entry into cardiac rehabilitation: a PILOT OBSERVATIONAL STUDY. J Cardiopulm Rehabil Prev. 2017;37(4):250–6.
33. Davies MJ, Gagliardino JJ, Gray LJ, Khunti K, Mohan V, Hughes R. Real-world factors affecting adherence to insulin therapy in patients with Type 1 or Type 2 diabetes mellitus: a systematic review. Diabet Med. 2013;30(5):512–24.
34. Manne JM, Snively CS, Ramsey JM, Salgado MO, Barnighausen T, Reich MR. Barriers to treatment access for Chagas disease in Mexico. PLoS Negl Trop Dis. 2013;7(10):e2488.
35. Baker DW. The meaning and the measure of health literacy. J Gen Intern Med. 2006;21(8):878–83.
36. Wolf MS, Davis TC, Osborn CY, Skripkauskas S, Bennett CL, Makoul G. Literacy, self-efficacy, and HIV medication adherence. Patient Educ Couns. 2007;65(2):253–60.
37. In: Nielsen-Bohlman L, Panzer AM, Kindig DA, editors. Health literacy: a prescription to end confusion. Washington DC: 2004 by the National Academy of Sciences; 2004.
38. Kutner M, Greenberg E, Jin Y, Paulsen C. The health literacy of America's adults: results from the 2003 National Assessment of Adult Literacy (NCES 2006-483). Washington, DC: U.S. Department of Education: National Center for Education Statistics; 2006.
39. Miller TA. Health literacy and adherence to medical treatment in chronic and acute illness: a meta-analysis. Patient Educ Couns. 2016;99(7):1079–86.
40. Brown MT, Bussell J, Dutta S, Davis K, Strong S, Mathew S. Medication adherence: truth and consequences. Am J Med Sci. 2016;351(4):387–99.
41. Hayward KL, Martin JH, Cottrell WN, Karmakar A, Horsfall LU, Patel PJ, et al. Patient-oriented education and medication management intervention for people with decompensated cirrhosis: study protocol for a randomized controlled trial. Trials. 2017;18(1):339.
42. Kobak KA, Taylor L, Katzelnick DJ, Olson N, Clagnaz P, Henk HJ. Antidepressant medication management and Health Plan Employer Data Information Set (HEDIS) criteria: reasons for nonadherence. J Clin Psychiatry. 2002;63(8):727–32.
43. Horne R, Weinman J. Patients' beliefs about prescribed medicines and their role in adherence to treatment in chronic physical illness. J Psychosom Res. 1999;47(6):555–67.
44. Horne R, Chapman SC, Parham R, Freemantle N, Forbes A, Cooper V. Understanding patients' adherence-related beliefs about medicines prescribed for long-term conditions: a meta-analytic review of the Necessity-Concerns Framework. PLoS One. 2013;8(12):e80633.
45. Galvan FH, Bogart LM, Wagner GJ, Klein DJ, Chen YT. Conceptualisations of masculinity and self-reported medication adherence among HIV-positive Latino men in Los Angeles, California, USA. Cult Health Sex. 2014;16(6):697–709.
46. Devaux S, Castela A, Archier E, Gallini A, Joly P, Misery L, et al. Adherence to topical treatment in psoriasis: a systematic literature review. J Eur Acad Dermatol Venereol. 2012;26(Suppl 3):61–7.
47. Winters A, Esse T, Bhansali A, Serna O, Mhatre S, Sansgiry S. Physician perception of patient medication adherence in a cohort of medicare advantage plans in Texas. J Manag Care Spec Pharm. 2016;22(3):305–12.
48. Lapane KL, Dube CE, Schneider KL, Quilliam BJ. Misperceptions of patients vs providers regarding medication-related communication issues. Am J Manag Care. 2007;13(11):613–8.
49. Linder LA, Wu YP, Macpherson CF, Fowler B, Wilson A, Jo Y, et al. Oral medication adherence among adolescents and young adults with cancer before and following use of a smartphone-based medication reminder app. J Adolesc Young Adult Oncol. 2018;8(2):122–30.

50. Butow P, Palmer S, Pai A, Goodenough B, Luckett T, King M. Review of adherence-related issues in adolescents and young adults with cancer. J Clin Oncol. 2010;28(32):4800–9.
51. Simons LE, McCormick ML, Mee LL, Blount RL. Parent and patient perspectives on barriers to medication adherence in adolescent transplant recipients. Pediatr Transplant. 2009;13(3):338–47.
52. Koster ES, Philbert D, de Vries TW, van Dijk L, Bouvy ML. "I just forget to take it": asthma self-management needs and preferences in adolescents. J Asthma. 2015;52(8):831–7.
53. Muluneh B, Deal A, Alexander MD, Keisler MD, Markey JM, Neal JM, et al. Patient perspectives on the barriers associated with medication adherence to oral chemotherapy. J Oncol Pharm Pract. 2018;24(2):98–109.
54. Jones-Caballero M, Pedrosa E, Penas PF. Self-reported adherence to treatment and quality of life in mild to moderate acne. Dermatology. 2008;217(4):309–14.
55. Goren A, Carter C, Lee S. Patient reported health outcomes and non-adherence in psoriasis patients receiving adalimumab or ustekinumab for moderate to severe plaque psoriasis. J Dermatolog Treat. 2016;27(1):43–50.
56. Pena-Robichaux V, Kvedar JC, Watson AJ. Text messages as a reminder aid and educational tool in adults and adolescents with atopic dermatitis: a pilot study. Dermatol Res Pract. 2010;2010:1–6.
57. Tarn DM, Flocke SA. New prescriptions: how well do patients remember important information? Fam Med. 2011;43(4):254–9.
58. Jansen J, Butow PN, van Weert JC, van Dulmen S, Devine RJ, Heeren TJ, et al. Does age really matter? Recall of information presented to newly referred patients with cancer. J Clin Oncol. 2008;26(33):5450–7.
59. Rork JF, Sheehan WJ, Gaffin JM, Timmons KG, Sidbury R, Schneider LC, et al. Parental response to written eczema action plans in children with eczema. Arch Dermatol. 2012;148(3):391–2.
60. Bloomberg J. Digital transformation moves pharma 'Beyond the Pill' 2014. Available from: https://www.forbes.com/sites/jasonbloomberg/2014/08/15/digital-transformation-moves-pharma-beyond-the-pill/#774a89ab1c58.
61. DiMatteo MR, Lepper HS, Croghan TW. Depression is a risk factor for noncompliance with medical treatment: meta-analysis of the effects of anxiety and depression on patient adherence. Arch Intern Med. 2000;160(14):2101–7.
62. Feldman SR, Zhao Y, Shi L, Tran MH. Economic and comorbidity burden among patients with moderate-to-severe psoriasis. J Manag Care Spec Pharm. 2015;21(10):874–88.
63. Kulkarni AS, Balkrishnan R, Camacho FT, Anderson RT, Feldman SR. Medication and health care service utilization related to depressive symptoms in older adults with psoriasis. J Drugs Dermatol. 2004;3(6):661–6.
64. Li Y, Zhou H, Cai B, Kahler KH, Tian H, Gabriel S, et al. Group-based trajectory modeling to assess adherence to biologics among patients with psoriasis. Clinicoecon Outcomes Res. 2014;6:197–208.
65. Miller IM, McAndrew RJ, Hamzavi I. Prevalence, risk factors, and comorbidities of hidradenitis suppurativa. Dermatol Clin. 2016;34(1):7–16.
66. Silverberg JI. Selected comorbidities of atopic dermatitis: atopy, neuropsychiatric, and musculoskeletal disorders. Clin Dermatol. 2017;35(4):360–6.
67. Holmes AD, Spoendlin J, Chien AL, Baldwin H, Chang ALS. Evidence-based update on rosacea comorbidities and their common physiologic pathways. J Am Acad Dermatol. 2018;78(1):156–66.
68. Patel N, Nadkarni A, Cardwell LA, Vera N, Frey C, Patel N, et al. Psoriasis, depression, and inflammatory overlap: a review. Am J Clin Dermatol. 2017;18(5):613–20.
69. Sin NL, DiMatteo MR. Depression treatment enhances adherence to antiretroviral therapy: a meta-analysis. Ann Behav Med. 2014;47(3):259–69.
70. Madden JM, Graves AJ, Ross-Degnan D, Briesacher BA, Soumerai SB. Cost-related medication nonadherence after implementation of Medicare Part D, 2006–2007. JAMA. 2009;302(16):1755–6.
71. Williams J, Steers WN, Ettner SL, Mangione CM, Duru OK. Cost-related nonadherence by medication type among Medicare Part D beneficiaries with diabetes. Med Care. 2013;51(2):193–8.
72. Blanchard J, Madden JM, Ross-Degnan D, Gresenz CR, Soumerai SB. The relationship between emergency department use and cost-related medication nonadherence among Medicare beneficiaries. Ann Emerg Med. 2013;62(5):475–85.
73. Harrold LR, Briesacher BA, Peterson D, Beard A, Madden J, Zhang F, et al. Cost-related medication nonadherence in older patients with rheumatoid arthritis. J Rheumatol. 2013;40(2):137–43.
74. Musich S, Cheng Y, Wang SS, Hommer CE, Hawkins K, Yeh CS. Pharmaceutical cost-saving strategies and their association with medication adherence in a Medicare Supplement Population. J Gen Intern Med. 2015;30(8):1208–14.
75. Zhang Y, Baik SH. Race/ethnicity, disability, and medication adherence among medicare beneficiaries with heart failure. J Gen Intern Med. 2014;29(4):602–7.
76. Balkrishnan R, Bhosle MJ, Camacho FT, Anderson RT. Predictors of medication adherence and associated health care costs in an older population with overactive bladder syndrome: a longitudinal cohort study. J Urol. 2006;175(3 Pt 1):1067–71; discussion 71–2.
77. Rolnick SJ, Pawloski PA, Hedblom BD, Asche SE, Bruzek RJ. Patient characteristics associated with medication adherence. Clin Med Res. 2013;11(2):54–65.

78. Goldman DP, Joyce GF, Zheng Y. Prescription drug cost sharing: associations with medication and medical utilization and spending and health. JAMA. 2007;298(1):61–9.
79. Gibson TB, Ozminkowski RJ, Goetzel RZ. The effects of prescription drug cost sharing: a review of the evidence. Am J Manag Care. 2005;11(11):730–40.
80. Austvoll-Dahlgren A, Aaserud M, Vist G, Ramsay C, Oxman AD, Sturm H, et al. Pharmaceutical policies: effects of cap and co-payment on rational drug use. Cochrane Database Syst Rev. 2008;1:CD007017.
81. Slota C, Davis SA, Blalock SJ, Carpenter DM, Muir KW, Robin AL, et al. Patient-physician communication on medication cost during Glaucoma visits. Optom Vis Sci. 2017;94(12):1095–101.
82. Lee IA, Maibach HI. Pharmionics in dermatology: a review of topical medication adherence. Am J Clin Dermatol. 2006;7(4):231–6.
83. Tan X, Feldman SR, Chang J, Balkrishnan R. Topical drug delivery systems in dermatology: a review of patient adherence issues. Expert Opin Drug Deliv. 2012;9(10):1263–71.
84. Shokeen D, O'Neill JL, Taheri A, Feldman SR. Are topical keratolytic agents needed in the treatment of scalp psoriasis? Dermatol Online J. 2014;20(3).
85. Feldman SR, Horn EJ, Balkrishnan R, Basra MK, Finlay AY, McCoy D, et al. Psoriasis: improving adherence to topical therapy. J Am Acad Dermatol. 2008;59(6):1009–16.

Chapter 2
Strategy to Monitor Adherence

Bernard Vrijens

Introduction

Outpatient drug therapy can be very cost-effective, but only when the drug itself is effective. Unfortunately, drug therapy failures are common and costly. Even for drugs with the highest cure rates, many patients fail to respond or only respond partially. This can cause multiple patient visits, trial courses with several different drugs and even hospitalisation. The only certain result of ineffective drug therapy is increased cost to the health care system [1].

The single most frequent cause of failed drug therapy is poor patient adherence to their prescribed regimen. The problem of non-adherence is well known since Hipocrates [2]. This long-neglected problem has been put into light by the WHO report in 2003 [3]; more than half of patients on long-term regimens fail to take prescribed medications correctly. But medication adherence problems are difficult to identify and treat, because patients with suboptimal adherence are tough to distinguish from truly nonresponsive patients. Nonadherence is also a problem when making critical dose level determinations and when titrating patients onto drug therapy. Poor adherence can lead to unnecessary testing, added therapy, and avoidable admissions.

Effective management of adherence can simplify clinical management and improve patient care, while at the same time minimizing negative outcomes and helping to lower total costs. The benefits of good adherence are particularly true with "crucial medications", drugs for which good patient adherence is essential to avoid serious negative therapeutic outcomes. Even for less crucial medications, good adherence equates with better, more cost-effective patient care. Patient adherence to medications requires special attention during the initiation of drug therapy, and it deserves support for effective long-term drug therapy. The WHO stated that "*Increasing the effectiveness of adherence interventions may have a far greater impact on the health of the population than any improvement in specific medical treatments*" [3]. Crucial to the study and management of any phenomenon, biomedical or otherwise, is the ability to make reliable and rich measurements.

B. Vrijens (✉)
AARDEX Group, The Labs, Liège Science Park, Liège, Belgium
e-mail: bernard.vrijens@aardexgroup.com

© Springer Nature Switzerland AG 2020
S. R. Feldman et al. (eds.), *Treatment Adherence in Dermatology*, Updates in Clinical Dermatology,
https://doi.org/10.1007/978-3-030-27809-0_2

The ABC Taxonomy for Medication Adherence

The ABC taxonomy defines the overarching concept of "*medication adherence*" as the process by which patients take their medication as prescribed and subdivides it into 3 interrelated yet distinct phases: initiation, implementation, and persistence [4].

(A) "*Initiation*"—when the patient takes the first dose of a prescribed medication—is typically a binary event (patients either start taking their medication or not in a given time period).

(B) "*Implementation*"—the extent to which a patient's actual dosing corresponds to the prescribed dosing regimen, from initiation until the last dose is taken—is a longitudinal description of patient behavior over time, i.e. their dosing history.

(C) "*Persistence*", —the time elapsed from initiation, until eventual treatment discontinuation (i.e. time to event); after discontinuation, a period of non-persistence may follow until the end of the prescribing period. (Fig. 2.1)

Non-adherence to medications can thus occur in the following situations or combinations thereof: late or non-initiation of the prescribed treatment, sub-optimal implementation of the dosing regimen or early discontinuation of the treatment. Over 700 determinants are associated to at least one element of non-adherence [5]. While often reported as statistically significant, their predictive value for an individual patient remains very poor [6].

In the field of dermatology, with numerous different skin conditions and a variety of therapies and treatment formulations/instructions, correct adherence to treatment is essential to obtaining optimal efficacy and safety outcomes [7].

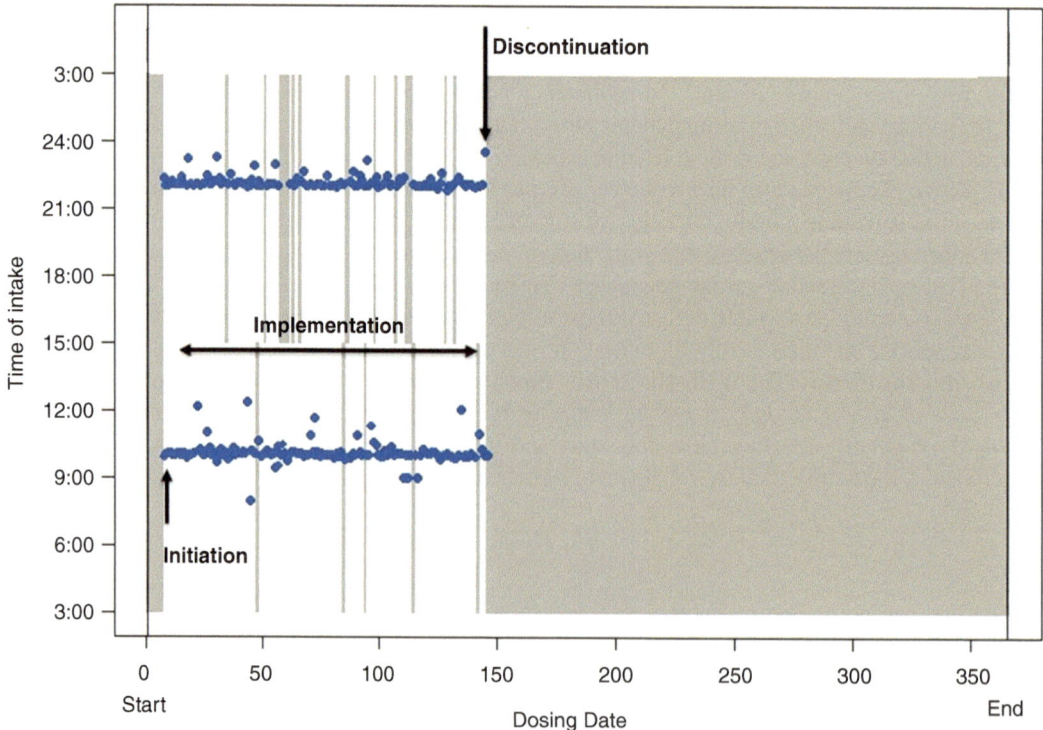

Fig. 2.1 Chronology plot of one case study to illustrate the taxonomy of medication adherence. Relative date from study start is shown on the horizontal axis, and 24-h clock time is shown on the vertical axis. Blue dots indicate the dates and times of drug intake. Grey bars indicate missed doses. Patient is on a twice-daily dosing regimen. The key elements of medication adherence are indicated with black arrows

Measurement of Medication Adherence

An apt quantification of adherence to medications constitutes the basis for sound adherence management.

Conventional methods for estimating missed doses, such as counting returned medications, or weighing returned cream tubes, don't indicate when doses are missed. More importantly, they are subject to upward bias by prevalent discarding or hoarding of untaken doses, i.e. some patients simply discard unused medications to please their study investigators or health carers. Clearly and self-evidently, any quantitative analysis that depends on human recall is *a priori* doomed to imprecision. It is doubtful that any individual could accurately recount information about the medication s/he took weeks prior, and further doubtful that s/he could recall what was forgotten.

Reliance on pill-count data or patient self-reported adherence is responsible for consistent overestimation and prevalent misunderstanding of patients' non-adherence in clinical trials and in medical practice.

Initiation and discontinuation of treatment are inherently discontinuous actions, whereas implementation of the dosing regimen is continuous. This difference precludes a single, quantitatively useful parameter to cover all three. For example, the four patients illustrated in Fig. 2.2 all took 81% of their prescribed one daily doses. However, the electronically compiled drug dosing history data reveal major differences in the dynamics of adherence to medications over time, which can reveal different causes and/or consequences.

Electronic Monitoring of Medication Adherence

The principle involved is called Medication Event Monitoring System (MEMS®), realized by incorporating microcircuitry into pharmaceutical packages of various design, such that the maneuvers needed to remove a dose of drug are detected, time-stamped, and stored. After being electronically captured in real time, drug dosing history data are validated as necessary, stored, and communicated. The drug dosing history can then be accessed for timely analysis and management of adherence to improve drug exposure and also support decision-making during drug development process [8] as well as in daily medical practice [9].

Electronic monitoring provides an objective record of a patient's actual dosing activity by recording the time and date of every opening of the drug package. Electronic detection of package entry is an indirect measure of dose intake and there could be instances where the package is activated but a dose is not taken. Studies comparing MEMS data with drug concentrations show that there is 97% accuracy between opening the pharmaceutical package and time of ingestion of the prescribed dose. This evidence advocates that MEMS packaging provides a very accurate measure of adherence and, even more importantly, insightful information of each individual's drug taking behaviors [8].

Electronic monitoring of patients' dosing histories has repeatedly revealed that the drug intake of ambulatory patients is frequently irregular, spanning a wide spectrum of deviations from the prescribed regimen. It is strongly skewed toward under-dosing, created by delayed and omitted doses, sometimes resulting in multiple, sequential omissions of prescribed doses. A major surprise has been the finding that life-threatening diseases do not, ipso facto, enforce strict execution of prescribed regimen(s). This fact became evident in the fields of organ transplantation [5, 10], HIV-AIDS [11], and more recently in oncology [12, 13].

Since the first published study based on MEMS in 1979, there have been over 800 peer-reviewed papers published describing clinical research that included use of MEMS in an aggregate population of over one million patients [14]. The principle of Medication Event Monitoring System has been

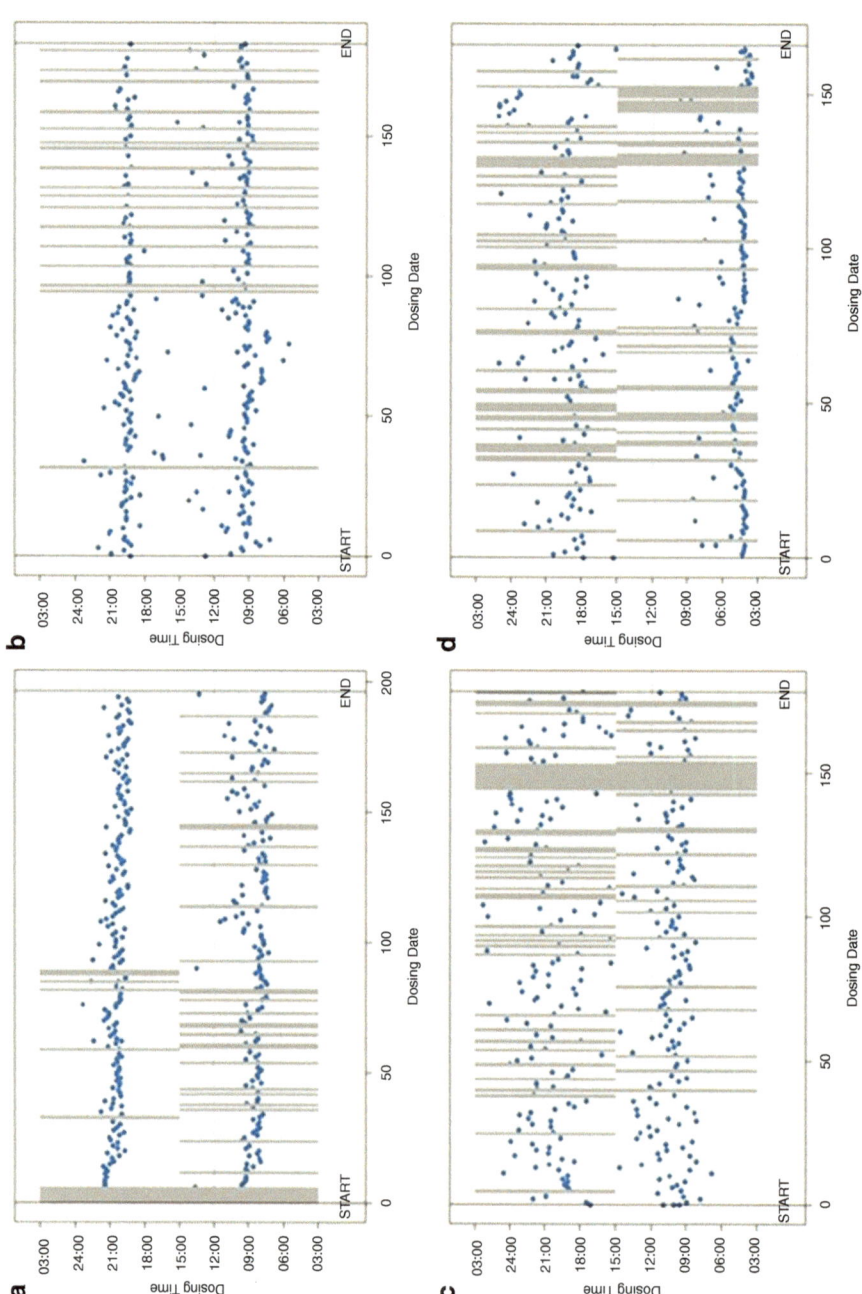

Fig. 2.2 Dosing chronology plots of four patients. Relative date from study start is shown on the horizontal axis, and 24-h clock time is shown on the vertical axis. Each blue dot indicates the electronically recorded time and date of dosing. The vertical tan lines depict missed doses. Extended periods without dosing (drug holidays) are shown by vertical tan bars, the width of which reflects the number of days without dosing. All 4 patients are on twice daily medication and have all taken 81% of their prescribed medications. Patient A delays treatment initiation by a few days and then implements the dosing regimen, missing primarily doses in the morning. Patient B takes timely the medication but after day 100, starts to skip regularly full days of treatment, primarily clustered on weekends. Patient C implements the dosing regimen with a wide variability in time of drug intake and missing primarily doses in the evening. Patient D implements with a low variability in time of intake in the morning and a wide variability in the evening

primarily used with bottle cap closure but also successfully applied to eye-drop dispensers, unit-dose blister packages, pump activations, syringe use, and the dispensing of creams and ointments from flexible tubes.

Management of Medication Adherence

Management of adherence is the process of monitoring and supporting patients' adherence to medications by health care systems, providers, patients, and their social networks. The objective of management of adherence is to achieve the best use by patients, of appropriately prescribed medicines, in order to maximize the potential for benefit and minimize the risk of harm [2].

Electronically-compiled dosing history data have been successfully used to support adherence-enhancing intervention, by allowing the health professional to provide feedback to the patient on his/her past dosing history. This approach has been referred to as "Measurement-Guided Medication Management (MGMM)" and is, thus, an approach to manage adherence to medications. Under this approach, reliable, detailed, recent, electronically-compiled drug dosing history data are provided as feedback to the patient on his/her adherence to prescribed medications. These data set the stage for focused dialogue between the health care team and their patients to reinforce behavioral, social, and cognitive interventions [15].

In this setting, there is a need for reliable data on patients' dosing histories to:

1. inform patients and caregivers when dosing errors have occurred;
2. suggest how best to minimize adverse consequences thereof;
3. reinforce each patient's understanding of the benefits, hazards, and limits of correct versus incorrect use of the medications they have been prescribed;
4. provide timely information on what to do when doses have been missed; and
5. reinforce information on the benefits of continued persistence with drugs prescribed for long-term use.

By reviewing the chronology plot and its derived analysis, the clinical team can identify adherence issues and share this information with the patient in order to identify and manage barriers that are compromising the optimal use of the treatment. It sets the stage for building a solid habit of medication taking [9].

Sound management of medication adherence makes it possible for the health care team to optimize patient adherence, improve care and lower costs. Electronic monitoring is an effective approach that provides objective data about a patient's record of self-dosing. This allows the clinical team and the patient to review the dosing record and work together to improve adherence.

The AARDEX Group's MEMS Adherence Software is a good example of a professional solution to present a comprehensive picture of patients' adherence using predefined and validated algorithms.

Adherence-Informed Prescriptions

For some patients, counseling and a review of the dosing record will effectively manage adherence and improve care. For other patients, electronically compiled data may lead the clinician to consider alternate therapies or other measures. For the entire patient population, clinical decisions are aided by objective data and resources are better allocated. Adherence-informed prescriptions enables the managed care provider to rapidly improve adherence, benefiting patients and lowering costs of care [16].

Conclusions

Imperfect medication adherence can limit the benefit of treatments, result in poorer outcomes for patients, and increase healthcare costs. Medication adherence can be decomposed into three distinct phases; (1) the initiation of treatment, (2) the degree to which a patient's dose taking matches the prescribed regimen (implementation) and (3) the discontinuation of treatment (persistence).

The wide range of drug dosing patterns that occurs among ambulatory patients is obscured by continued use of unreliable methods that afford patients the easy ability to censor evidence of omitted doses (*e.g.,* returned tablet counts, blood sampling, interviews, questionnaires, diaries) or methods that put unrealistic burden on patients' recall of past events.

The pervasive use of returned tablet/capsule counts for drug accountability in clinical trials has perpetuated the false notion that patient adherence in clinical trials is "good". Collectively, the >800 peer-reviewed papers based on smart packages have had a substantial impact on current views about patient adherence and its management. These views are strikingly different from what is typically reported from clinical trials.

Smart Packages allow automatic compilation of drug dosing history, which is the natural input to pharmacometric models of pharmacokinetic and pharmacodynamic responses to prescribed regimens of drug administration, however well or poorly adhered to. In addition to its pharmacometric role, the electronically-compiled drug dosing history is the logical foundation for the emerging method of measurement-guided management of prescribed (or protocol-specified) dosing regimens, aimed at achieving and maintaining correct adherence to prescribed drug dosing regimens.

MEMS reads and transfers stored dosing records, analyzes the data, and generates a variety of reports that detail or summarize patient dosing information. It is a valuable tool for monitoring crucial medicines in patients for whom adherence can have serious medical and economic consequences. For merit-based incentive payment system and pay for performance programs, this translates into more cost/effective treatment better control of health care costs and improved patient outcomes.

References

1. Khan R, Socha-Dietrich K. Investing in medication adherence improves health outcomes and health system efficiency: Adherence to medicines for diabetes, hypertension, and hyperlipidaemia. OECD Health Working Paper; 2018.
2. Vrijens B, De Geest S, Hughes DA, Przemyslaw K, Demonceau J, Ruppar T, et al. A new taxonomy for describing and defining adherence to medications. Br J Clin Pharmacol. 2012;73(5):691–705.
3. WHO. Adherence to long-term therapies: evidence for action. Geneva, Switzerland: World Health Organization; 2003.
4. De Geest S, Zullig LL, Dunbar-Jacob J, Helmy R, Hughes DA, Wilson IB, et al. ESPACOMP medication adherence reporting guideline (EMERGE). Ann Intern Med. 2018;169(1):30–5.
5. De Geest S, Moons P, Dobbels F, Martin S, Vanhaecke J. Profiles of patients who experienced a late acute rejection due to nonadherence with immunosuppressive therapy. J Cardiovasc Nurs. 2001;16(1):1–14.
6. Kardas P, Lewek P, Matyjaszczyk M. Determinants of patient adherence: a review of systematic reviews. Front Pharmacol. 2013;4:91.
7. Feldman SR, Vrijens B, Gieler U, Piaserico S, Puig L, van de Kerkhof P. Treatment adherence intervention studies in dermatology and guidance on how to support adherence. Am J Clin Dermatol. 2017;18(2):253–71.
8. Vrijens B, Urquhart J. Methods for measuring, enhancing, and accounting for medication adherence in clinical trials. Clin Pharmacol Ther. 2014;95(6):617–26.
9. Vrijens B, Urquhart J, White D. Electronically monitored dosing histories can be used to develop a medication-taking habit and manage patient adherence. Expert Rev Clin Pharmacol. 2014;7(5):633–44.
10. Nevins TE, Kruse L, Skeans MA, Thomas W. The natural history of azathioprine compliance after renal transplantation. Kidney Int. 2001;60(4):1565–70.
11. Paterson DL, Swindells S, Mohr J, Brester M, Vergis EN, Squier C, et al. Adherence to protease inhibitor therapy and outcomes in patients with HIV infection. Ann Intern Med. 2000;133(1):21–30.

12. Marin D, Bazeos A, Mahon FX, Eliasson L, Milojkovic D, Bua M, et al. Adherence is the critical factor for achieving molecular responses in patients with chronic myeloid leukemia who achieve complete cytogenetic responses on imatinib. J Clin Oncol. 2010;28(14):2381–8.

13. Bhatia S, Landier W, Hageman L, Kim H, Chen Y, Crews KR, et al. 6MP adherence in a multiracial cohort of children with acute lymphoblastic leukemia: a Children's Oncology Group Study. Blood. 2014;124(15):2345–53.

14. https://iadherence.aardexgroup.com/iadherence-ref-spring/biblio/index.htm. Last update: February 1, 2019.

15. Demonceau J, Ruppar T, Kristanto P, Hughes DA, et al. Identification and assessment of adherence enhancing interventions in studies assessing medication adherence through electronically compiled drug dosing histories: a systematic literature review and meta-analysis. Accepted for publication in Drugs 2013 (Manuscript number: DRUA-D-13-00032R1).

16. Hughes D. When drugs don't work: economic assessment of enhancing compliance with interventions supported by electronic monitoring devices. PharmacoEconomics. 2007;25(8):621–35.

Chapter 3
Strategies to Improve Adherence

Sree S. Kolli, Adrian Pona, Abigail Cline, and Steven R. Feldman

Introduction

A good patient-physician relationship is integral to optimizing adherence to treatment and clinical outcomes. However, the concept of the patient-physician relationship has been evolving in recent years. Previously, an asymmetric relationship between the physician and the patient was assumed – the physician knows best about the disease and treatment, the patient accepts this and follows instructions. In this model, the term compliance described the patient's consent to follow medical recommendation. Compliance implies that the physician instructs and the patient is to follow those instructions. Recently, the patient-physician relationship has become viewed as a more collaborative process, one which the patient is more involved in the decision process. For this reason, the term adherence has replaced compliance and the even newer term concordance has been proposed [1]. Concordance more clearly implies a shared responsibility between the physician and patient to agree on medical recommendations.

The realization has also arisen that adherence does not rest alone with the patient. Other factors— such as the physician, the diagnosis, and the medication— may influence the patient's adherence behavior. Patients may accept or reject the medical advice, especially depending on the relationship they have with their physician. A growing body of literature supports the positive effect of agreement within the patient-physician relationship on adherence and patient outcomes [2]. Other studies demonstrate that disagreements between patients and physicians lead to poor adherence and health outcomes [3, 4]. For this reason, it may be helpful to understand how physicians can influence agreement, and ultimately patients' adherence to treatment.

There are many aspects of the patient-physician relationship for which physicians have some degree of direct control. These include continuity of care, patients' trust in their physician, and the ability of the physician to enable the patient toward effective self-management. Physicians build trust by creating a supportive and friendly environment that eases patients' distress. By educating

S. S. Kolli · A. Pona (✉) · A. Cline
Department of Dermatology, Wake Forest School of Medicine, Winston-Salem, NC, USA
e-mail: apona@wakehealth.edu

S. R. Feldman
Departments of Dermatology, Pathology and Social Sciences & Health Policy, Wake Forest School of Medicine, Winston-Salem, NC, USA

© Springer Nature Switzerland AG 2020
S. R. Feldman et al. (eds.), *Treatment Adherence in Dermatology*, Updates in Clinical Dermatology, https://doi.org/10.1007/978-3-030-27809-0_3

patients on the disease and treatment plan, physicians increase patient confidence patients have in their physician, in their treatment regimen, and in their own self-management. In addition to building trust in the physician and confidence with simple interventions, physicians may employ more advanced strategies to develop agreement with the patient on the recommended treatment plan. This chapter will examine interventions ranging from basic interventions to more complex techniques to improve patient adherence.

Physician-Centered Strategies

There are three levels of physician-centered strategies, which can be viewed as a pyramid (Fig. 3.1). The first level is the foundation which consists of developing a strong patient-physician relationship of trust and building a sense of accountability. The next level relies on standard interventions in areas such as cost, simple treatment regimens, patient education to foster adherence; without the foundation, however, these interventions should not be expected to be very effective. The final level involves more advanced psychological techniques that help foster agreement between the patient and the physician about the recommended treatment plan.

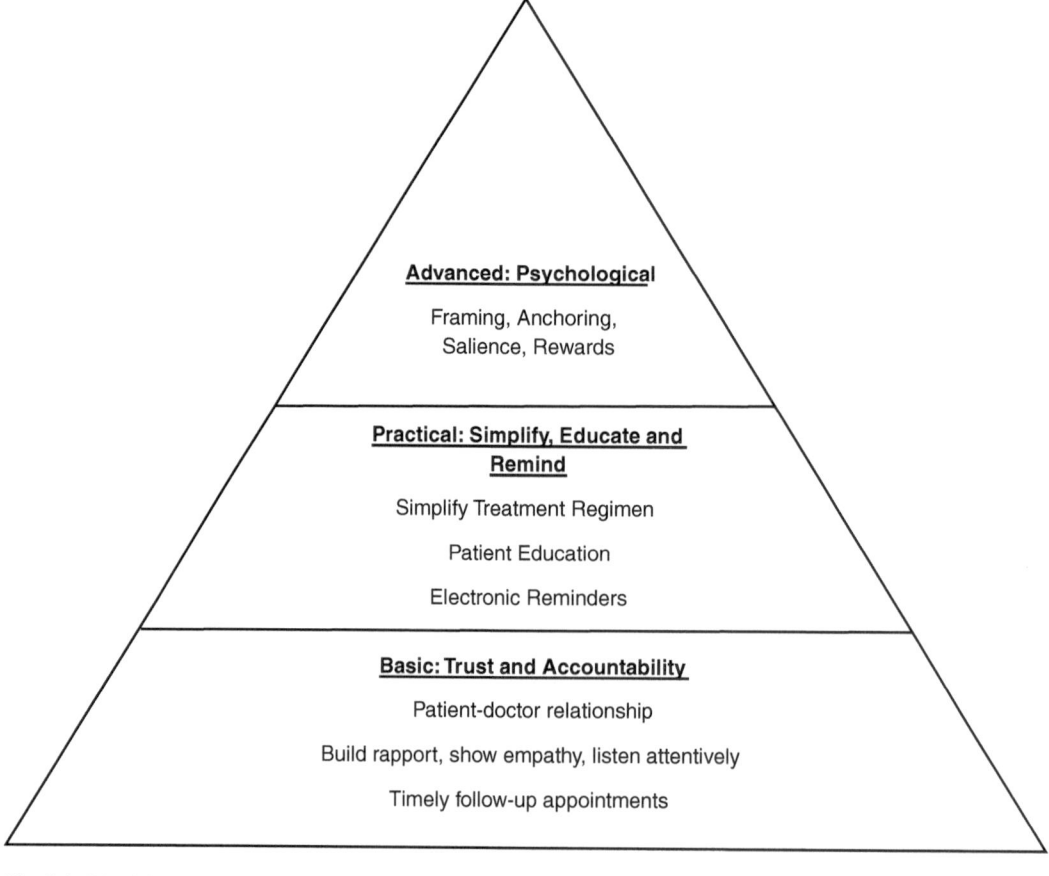

Fig. 3.1 Physician-centered strategies

Foundation: Trust and Accountability

An important step to improving adherence is building a foundation that increases trust and accountability. Trust develops over time as physicians build rapport with patients, create a friendly, supportive environment, and appear understanding to patients' situations and concerns. Being perceived as a caring physician is central to building this trust. A physician's interpersonal skills such as showing empathy, listening attentively and clear communication are important in fostering trust, allowing patients to reveal any barriers affecting their ability to take their medications [5]. Studies on the doctor-patient relationship focus on how these interpersonal skills rather than time spent can lead to increased satisfaction of care [6, 7]. Increased patient satisfaction with the doctor-patient relationship improves treatment adherence [8]. In pediatric atopic dermatitis (AD), the strongest predictor of adherence to skincare advice is a solid doctor-patient or caregiver relationship. This results in greater self-efficacy as mothers feel more comfortable managing their children's disease [9]. For psoriasis patients using biologics, patient-physician communication and good interpersonal relations were drivers for greater adherence [10].

Another important component at this level is improving accountability by scheduling an early follow up visit or other contact with the patient. Early and frequent follow-up visits increases the likelihood of patients taking their medication in anticipation of those visits with the physician [11, 12]. An analysis of 5 studies on AD patients and adherence revealed that the length of time between baseline and first return visit was inversely proportional to adherence [13].

Practical: Simplify, Educate, and Remind

After establishing a foundation, the next level of physician-centered strategies involves simple, effective interventions that physicians can implement to help patients manage their conditions better. This includes simplifying treatment regimens, patient education, medication reminders, and medication cost.

Simplified Treatment Regimens and Patient Preference

Overly complicated treatment regimens are common impediments to poor adherence. Although multiple treatments might be effective in improving outcomes if they were all used, the complexity of such regimens increase treatment burden, may reduce adherence, and, potentially, worsen treatment outcomes. When multiple treatments are needed, simplifying the treatment regimens by prescribing a combination product with multiple active ingredients may be a worthwhile intervention. A clinical trial randomized 26 subjects with mild-to-moderate acne to clindamycin phosphate 1.2%-tretinoin 0.025% (CTG) gel or clindamycin phosphate 1% gel plus tretinoin 0.025% cream (C gel + T cream) for 12 weeks. At week 12, the median adherence of the combination group was higher than for the group that received C gel + T cream separately (86% vs 14%, $P = 0.02$) [14].

Patients may prefer one treatment over another, the vehicle type of a medication, or a certain dosing schedule that is convenient for them. Messy application is a common reason for nonadherence so patients may prefer less greasy topical corticosteroid vehicles such as foams or sprays [15]. About 69% of patients using biologics preferred a less frequent dosing schedule limited to once every 12 weeks as opposed to 1-week or 2-week dosing schedules [16]. It is important for physicians to listen to these patient preferences and adjust care because patients feel more empowered when they help develop the treatment plan and thus are more likely to adhere to it [17].

Patient Education

Educating patients is a simple intervention that can be done during the clinic office visit, sometimes with the aid of technology or through formalized workshops. The impact of education on adherence can be considerable as patients learn more about the disease and treatments and may influence patients' perceptions of treatment efficacy and necessity. Educating patients during the office visit is effective as patients respond better when they receive individualized advice and learn how to incorporate management into everyday lives [18]. However, this may be more time consuming and results in less recall by patients if the information is presented verbally with no other educational aids [19, 20].

Written information in the form of written action plans, pamphlets, and office posters are useful tools to aid in relaying vital information to patients. Providing written information can also save time and be cost effective. Lists are more effective than paragraphs [21, 22]. Written information along with verbal instructions can help with recall [23]. Individualized printed materials tailored to patient's demographics and stage of disease are more likely to be read than general information about the disease [24]. A multidisciplinary, informative brochure plus a personalized patient notebook can teach patients on how to manage their disease and result in improved quality of life and severity of disease [25].

The use of audiotapes, videotapes, computer-assisted patient education can assist physicians in teaching patients. These modes of information are more interactive and may help reduce the amount of time physicians have to spend educating and addressing patient concerns and questions. In addition, the use of the internet in educating patients may be effective if patients are directed to the right resources. For example, the Contact Allergen Replacement Database is a fabulous resource that allows dermatologists to input allergens and develop lists of products free of those allergens and saves time patients searching for the appropriate products [14]. The National Psoriasis Foundation offers a host of brochures on treatment options that can be used to educate patients on the risks, benefits and alternatives of commonly used systemic treatments for psoriasis.

Regardless of the mode of education, educating can have a substantial impact on helping patients manage their disease and improve adherence. A multicenter, clinical trial randomized 97 subjects with acne to either adapalene/benzoyl peroxide (A/BPO) + supplementary education material (SEM), A/BPO + 2 additional visits or A/BPO alone. A/BPO + SEM group had more subjects with greater than 75% adherence compared to A/BPO+ 2 additional visits and A/BPO alone groups (45% vs 30.4% vs 25%), although mean adherence was still less than 50% in all groups [26]. The impact of oral and written counseling on treatment adherence in acne patients was assessed by randomizing 80 subjects to receive either a patient information leaflet plus oral instruction via telephone or oral counseling during the clinic visit only. There was a higher self-reported adherence in the group that received oral and written instruction compared to group with standard office visit instructions (80% vs 62%, $P = 0.043$) [27].

Medication Reminders

Timely reminders can be another simple intervention physicians can utilize in helping improve adherence. Text message reminders are a novel way to improve adherence and convenient for patients to use. Daily text message reminders were sent to 20 patients with psoriasis for 12 weeks. Adherence was measured by investigating how many days per week patients correctly took their medication. At Week 12, the daily text message intervention group had a 67.4% increase in adherence from baseline (adherence improved from 3.86 days/week to 6.46 days/week; $P < 0.001$) [28]. Another way to incorporate reminders is to use a smartphone app that has built in reminders that pop up on screen. A clinical trial randomized 134 psoriasis subjects treated with once-daily calcipotriol/betamethasone dipropionate (Cal/BD) foam to receive either a smartphone app reminder or standard care. Subjects who used the app were much more adherent to Cal/BD foam than were subjects in the control group (65% vs 38%, $P = 0.004$) at Week 4 [29].

Cost

Unaffordable drug prices may negatively impact adherence. Healthcare providers can prescribe low-cost generic medications to help reduce the burden of treatment. Furthermore, providers may also communicate with pharmacies to choose the best cost-effective treatment for the patient. Although brand name medications are generally more expensive then generic, some generic medications may also be expensive. Therefore, choosing the most cost-effective medication in a collaborative approach between the healthcare provider, patient, and pharmacy, could avoid a detrimental impact on the patient economically [30].

Advanced: Psychological Techniques

Physicians may employ a variety of psychological techniques including framing, anchoring, salience and rewards when discussing potential treatment recommendations with patients to increase the likelihood that patients will adhere.

Framing

Framing the information patients receive may influence their perspective on the treatment. Framing is a type of cognitive bias in which people react to a particular choice in different ways depending on how it is presented. Many times, patients may fear the adverse effects (AEs) of a given medication, and framing the information about AEs can help lessen those fears. For example, if a medication has a 1/1000 chance of causing AEs, a physician could frame this piece of information by saying that 999/1000 people using the medication do not experience AEs. Patients fine the latter framing—999 out of 1000 not having an AE—more reassuring even though the two approaches are mathematically identical ways of presenting the information. One study analyzed the different ways in which information on actinic keratosis (AK) was presented and how that influenced whether patients sought treatment. Of the patients who were told AKs were precancerous, 92.2% preferred treatment [31]. Of patients who were told AKs do not progress to cancer, 57.7% chose treatment [31].

Another way to reduce the negative effects of AEs on adherence is to explain to patients that AEs are signs that a medication is working. Some patients might stop the medication if they experience pain or burning after applying a topical agent. If patients are told beforehand that these AEs are indicators that a medication is working (and arguably such side effects are a sign the medication is working because these side effects indicate the patient is effectively applying the medication), patients may be more likely to continue with the medication instead of prematurely stop it. Framing the same information in a different way is a powerful tool to change a patient's perspective and influence their decision on treatment.

Anchoring

Anchoring can reduce the perceived burden of treatment. Anchoring occurs when people make a judgment relative to the first piece of information. For example, if patients are presented a complex, difficult dosing regimen first, they may find a standard regimen more appealing. In the treatment of psoriasis patients who've never before taken by injection but who need a biologic, it may be helpful to explain that, "biologics have to be taken like insulin: by injection. You know how diabetics have to take insulin injections twice a day? Well, this medication is a lot like that, only you don't have to take it twice a day, you only need to take it once a month." If patients are simply offered once a month injections, they mentally compare taking a shot once a month to not taking shots, and it doesn't seem very appealing. On the other hand, if patients are first anchored on the idea of shots twice a day, the 1 month frequency of injection seems very tolerable. One study measured this anchoring technique with biologics, and patients anchored to once-daily injectable biologic intervention were more willing (on a scale of 1–10) to start a once-monthly injectable biologic (median, 7.5) than those not anchored to a once-daily injection first (median, 2.0, $P < 0.001$) [32]. Anchoring can dramatically change the perception of treatment, making a standard approach seem like a bargain compared to a less appealing dosage regimen.

Salience

Salience relies on creating a vivid picture in a patient's mind that may make patients more amendable to a treatment. Presenting quantitative statistics about the effects of a treatment may not be as attention-grabbing as creating a picture or presenting an anecdote that is more likely to stick in patients' minds. For example, explaining that 9 out of 10 psoriasis patient clear up with a topical corticosteroid may seem promising to patients, but it may not be as powerful as creating a visual image. If a physician described how a psoriasis patient with large erythematous, scaly plaques all over their body cleared up with consistent use of a topical corticosteroid, started wearing a two-piece bathing suit, and wore a sleeveless wedding dress, patients may be more willing to try the same treatment compared to a physician who provides statistical facts about the treatment.

Reward System

A final technique that can be used is a rewards system to improve adherence. This technique draws from the psychological idea of operant condition and positive reinforcement. Adding a positive, reinforcing stimulus following a behavior will increase the chance the behavior will occur again in the future. A sticker calendar chart can be a tool for rewarding children with AD when they take their medication. A sticker is placed on each day of the calendar following a dose administration which provides positive reinforcement as well as a reminder for the next dose of medication.

Conclusion

Each of three levels of physician-centered strategies target different areas to help improve adherence. The foundation level focuses on improving the patient-doctor relationship and establishing accountability; without these, other approaches are likely not to be particularly effective. Once this foundation is established, specific approaches can be used to address the common reasons cited for nonadherence; belief in treatment inefficacy and forgetfulness may be overcome with education and medication reminders. More advanced psychological techniques— such as framing the efficacy of treatment more positively and reducing disproportionate concerns about adverse effects—are among a host of other approaches physicians can use to enhance adherence and treatment outcomes.

Conflicts of Interest Dr. Steven Feldman has received research, speaking and/or consulting support from a variety of companies including Galderma, GSK/Stiefel, Almirall, Leo Pharma, Boehringer Ingelheim, Mylan, Celgene, Pfizer, Valeant, Abbvie, Samsung, Janssen, Lilly, Menlo, Merck, Novartis, Regeneron, Sanofi, Novan, Qurient, National Biological Corporation, Caremark, Advance Medical, Sun Pharma, Suncare Research, Informa, UpToDate and National Psoriasis Foundation. He is founder and majority owner of www.DrScore.com and founder and part owner of Causa Research, a company dedicated to enhancing patients' adherence to treatment.

Dr. Adrian Pona, Dr. Abigail Cline, and Sree S. Kolli has no conflicts to disclose.

References

1. Taube KM. Patient-doctor relationship in dermatology: from compliance to concordance. Acta Derm Venereol. 2016;96(217):25–9.
2. Dwamena F, Holmes-Rovner M, Gaulden CM, Jorgenson S, Sadigh G, Sikorskii A, et al. Interventions for providers to promote a patient-centred approach in clinical consultations. Cochrane Database Syst Rev. 2012;12:CD003267.
3. Peikes D, Zutshi A, Genevro JL, Parchman ML, Meyers DS. Early evaluations of the medical home: building on a promising start. Am J Manag Care. 2012;18(2):105–16.
4. Rathert C, Wyrwich MD, Boren SA. Patient-centered care and outcomes: a systematic review of the literature. Med Care Res Rev. 2013;70(4):351–79.
5. Dorr Goold S, Lipkin M Jr. The doctor-patient relationship: challenges, opportunities, and strategies. J Gen Intern Med. 1999;14(Suppl 1):S26–33.
6. Feldman SR. Approaching psoriasis differently: patient-physician relationships, patient education and choosing the right topical vehicle. J Drugs Dermatol. 2010;9(8):908–11.
7. Renzi C, Abeni D, Picardi A, Agostini E, Melchi CF, Pasquini P, et al. Factors associated with patient satisfaction with care among dermatological outpatients. Br J Dermatol. 2001;145(4):617–23.
8. Harris DR. The art of treating psoriasis: practical suggestions for improved treatment. Cutis. 1999;64(5):335–6.
9. Ohya Y, Williams H, Steptoe A, Saito H, Iikura Y, Anderson R, et al. Psychosocial factors and adherence to treatment advice in childhood atopic dermatitis. J Invest Dermatol. 2001;117(4):852–7.
10. Zschocke I, Ortland C, Reich K. Evaluation of adherence predictors for the treatment of moderate to severe psoriasis with biologics: the importance of physician-patient interaction and communication. J Eur Acad Dermatol Venereol. 2017;31(6):1014–20.
11. Sagransky MJ, Yentzer BA, Williams LL, Clark AR, Taylor SL, Feldman SR. A randomized controlled pilot study of the effects of an extra office visit on adherence and outcomes in atopic dermatitis. Arch Dermatol. 2010;146(12):1428–30.
12. Davis SA, Lin HC, Yu CH, Balkrishnan R, Feldman SR. Underuse of early follow-up visits: a missed opportunity to improve patients' adherence. J Drugs Dermatol. 2014;13(7):833–6.
13. Shah A, Yentzer BA, Feldman SR. Timing of return office visit affects adherence to topical treatment in patients with atopic dermatitis: an analysis of 5 studies. Cutis. 2013;91(2):105–7.
14. Yentzer BA, Ade RA, Fountain JM, Clark AR, Taylor SL, Fleischer AB Jr, et al. Simplifying regimens promotes greater adherence and outcomes with topical acne medications: a randomized controlled trial. Cutis. 2010;86(2):103–8.
15. Brown KK, Rehmus WE, Kimball AB. Determining the relative importance of patient motivations for nonadherence to topical corticosteroid therapy in psoriasis. J Am Acad Dermatol. 2006;55(4):607–13.
16. Zhang M, Carter C, Olson WH, Johnson MP, Brennem SK, Lee S, et al. Patient preference for dosing frequency based on prior biologic experience. J Drugs Dermatol. 2017;16(3):220–6.
17. Moradi Tuchayi S, Alexander TM, Nadkarni A, Feldman SR. Interventions to increase adherence to acne treatment. Patient Prefer Adherence. 2016;10:2091–6.
18. Krakowski AC, Eichenfield LF, Dohil MA. Management of atopic dermatitis in the pediatric population. Pediatrics. 2008;122(4):812–24.
19. Kongsted A, Qerama E, Kasch H, Bach FW, Korsholm L, Jensen TS, et al. Education of patients after whiplash injury: is oral advice any better than a pamphlet? Spine. 2008;33(22):E843–8.
20. Vanderberg-Dent S. Part II. Challenges in educating patients. Dis Mon. 2000;46(12):798–810.
21. Dimou C. Patient education. Part III. Patient compliance. Dis Mon. 2000;46(12):811–22.
22. Morrow DG, Leirer VO, Andrassy JM, Hier CM, Menard WE. The influence of list format and category headers on age differences in understanding medication instructions. Exp Aging Res. 1998;24(3):231–56.
23. Isaacman DJ, Purvis K, Gyuro J, Anderson Y, Smith D. Standardized instructions: do they improve communication of discharge information from the emergency department? Pediatrics. 1992;89(6 Pt 2):1204–8.
24. Skinner CS, Campbell MK, Rimer BK, Curry S, Prochaska JO. How effective is tailored print communication? Ann Behav Med. 1999;21(4):290–8.
25. Tschopp JM, Frey JG, Janssens JP, Burrus C, Garrone S, Pernet R, et al. Asthma outpatient education by multiple implementation strategy. Outcome of a programme using a personal notebook. Respir Med. 2005;99(3):355–62.
26. Myhill T, Coulson W, Nixon P, Royal S, McCormack T, Kerrouche N. Use of supplementary patient education material increases treatment adherence and satisfaction among acne patients receiving adapalene 0.1%/benzoyl peroxide 2.5% gel in primary care clinics: a multicenter, randomized, controlled clinical study. Dermatol Ther. 2017;7(4):515–24.
27. Navarrete-Dechent C, Curi-Tuma M, Nicklas C, Cardenas C, Perez-Cotapos ML, Salomone C. Oral and written counseling is a useful instrument to improve short-term adherence to treatment in acne patients: a randomized controlled trial. Dermatol Pract Concept. 2015;5(4):13–6.

28. Balato N, Megna M, Di Costanzo L, Balato A, Ayala F. Educational and motivational support service: a pilot study for mobile-phone-based interventions in patients with psoriasis. Br J Dermatol. 2013;168(1):201–5.

29. Svendsen MT, Andersen F, Andersen KH, Pottegard A, Johannessen H, Moller S, et al. A smartphone application supporting patients with psoriasis improves adherence to topical treatment: a randomized controlled trial. Br J Dermatol. 2018;179(5):1062–71.

30. Lewis DJ, Feldman, SR. Practical ways to improve patient adherence. Columbia, SC: CreateSpace Independent Publishing Platform. 2017.

31. Berry K, Butt M, Kirby JS. Influence of information framing on patient decisions to treat actinic keratosis. JAMA Dermatol. 2017;153(5):421–6.

32. Oussedik E, Cardwell LA, Patel NU, Onikoyi O, Feldman SR. An anchoring-based intervention to increase patient willingness to use injectable medication in psoriasis. JAMA Dermatol. 2017;153(9):932–4.

Chapter 4
Psychological Techniques to Promote Adherence

Monica Shah, Felicia Tai, Abigail Cline, Adrian Pona, E. J. Masicampo, and Steven R. Feldman

Introduction

Providers often assume that the patient is capable of following a treatment regimen. However, research reveals this assumption to be erroneous. The lack of concordance between patient readiness and practitioner recommendations means that treatments are frequently offered to patients who are not ready to follow them. This reflects a bias towards treating the medical problem and underestimating the behavioral requirements of the treatment regimen.

Adherence is a complex behavioral process involving several interacting factors. These include characteristics of the patient, the patient's environment (such as social supports, understanding of the health care system, functioning of the health care team, and accessibility to health care resources), and features of the disease in question and its treatment. Psychology offers useful theories, models, and strategies that supports evidence-based approaches to promoting adherence. Adherence interventions based on behavioral principles has been demonstrated in areas such as cancer, asthma, diabetes, and even sun-protection [1–4]. Psychological techniques can also be applied to health care providers and health care systems [5, 6].

This chapter describes several traits that are behavioral in nature and are also dynamic, and therefore amenable to intervention. We will discuss basic psychological principles of patients, health care providers, and health systems, and models of behavioral change that are relevant to adherence to treatment for dermatological conditions.

M. Shah · F. Tai
Faculty of Medicine, University of Toronto, Toronto, ON, Canada

A. Cline · A. Pona (✉)
Department of Dermatology, Wake Forest School of Medicine, Winston-Salem, NC, USA
e-mail: apona@wakehealth.edu

E. J. Masicampo
Department of Psychology, Wake Forest University, Winston-Salem, NC, USA

S. R. Feldman
Departments of Dermatology, Pathology and Social Sciences & Health Policy, Wake Forest School of Medicine, Winston-Salem, NC, USA

© Springer Nature Switzerland AG 2020
S. R. Feldman et al. (eds.), *Treatment Adherence in Dermatology*, Updates in Clinical Dermatology,
https://doi.org/10.1007/978-3-030-27809-0_4

Patient-Centered Approaches

A patient's attitudes, beliefs, and choices can prevent that patient from following treatment recommendations. Patient-based psychological approaches involve patients learning by association, such as developing self-management techniques, or learning how particular behaviors associate with a health outcome, such as cognitive behavioral therapy. Other techniques discussed in this section include adopting healthier coping-mechanisms, fostering self-efficacy, building self-awareness, and attending support groups.

Coping-Mechanisms

Coping mechanisms are psychological processes developed at a conscious level to manage difficult and stressful situations. The precipitation of adverse events and the subsequent coping mechanisms are known to mitigate adherent behaviour. For example, the consumption of alcohol may often be used as a coping mechanism for the patients dealing with distressing dermatologic disorders [7]. However, alcohol usage is associated with nonadherence in conditions such as atopic dermatitis, actinic keratosis, and acne [8–10]. In actinic keratosis, alcohol consumption negatively correlates with treatment satisfaction relating to the side effects of field therapy [9]. Furthermore, a study on subjects being treated for atopic dermatitis found that alcohol intake of greater than once a month was correlated with decreased adherence for oral medications, but not topical treatments [8].

Coping styles may be adaptive (meaning that the individual tries to reduce the stress) or maladaptive (meaning the individual keeps or even amplifies the current stressor). Examples of coping styles include: problem-focused coping, which includes planning, active approach, and deletion of concurrent activities; emotion-focused coping, which includes positive interpretation and growth, restraint, and acceptance; social support-focused coping, which includes the use of the social–instrumental support, the use of the social–emotional support, and the expression of feelings (venting of emotions); and avoidant coping, which includes denial and both mental and behavioral deactivation [11].

The relationship between different coping styles and dermatological patients has been explored in conditions such as melanoma, hidradenitis suppurativa (HS), and psoriasis [12–14]. Overall, patients with problem-focused coping had better adjustment to melanoma than those with passive or avoidant coping. Additionally, patients with problem-focused coping reported higher levels of self-esteem and vigor, fewer physical symptoms, and less anger and fatigue. In contrast, avoidance coping is associated with anxiety, depression, confusion, and mood disturbance in patients with early-stage melanoma [15]. Patients with HS utilized several coping and social support strategies, including positive reframing, humor, social-support, and avoidance [13]. Psoriasis patients who more frequently used normalizing/optimistic coping reported higher levels of mental health while those that used combined emotive coping strategies reported more disability, poorer mental health, and worse overall quality of life [14].

Although the relationship between coping mechanisms and adherence has not yet been explored for dermatological conditions, different coping mechanisms are associated with improved or worse adherence in other chronic diseases, such as chronic obstructive pulmonary disease (COPD) and diabetes mellitus [16, 17]. In a study of patients with COPD, the depression score was the highest in patients with avoidance-type coping and the lowest in patients with problem-focused coping (11.0 vs 5.6; $P = 0.042$), respectively, patients with social support-focused coping having the highest anxiety score in contrast to patients with emotion-focused coping, which had the lowest anxiety score (11.6 vs 5.0; $P = 0.006$) [16]. In diabetic patients, patients with emotion-focused coping had the highest level ($P = 0.02$) of diabetes-related self-care activities, followed by patients with social support-focused coping, and problem-focused coping, while patients with avoidance-focused coping had the lowest total score. Furthermore, patients with emotion-focused and social support-focused coping styles had increased adherence to diabetes-related self-care activities, while patients with other dominant coping styles were less interested in managing their disease [17].

In case of a multidisciplinary approach, identifying the coping styles in patients with chronic dermatological diseases represents an important aspect of the individualized treatment of the patient. While research suggests that people with more adaptive coping styles may have better adherence, it remains uncertain whether certain coping styles truly have a causal effect on adherence. For those with avoidant or social support-focused coping, psychological intervention such as cognitive behavior therapy may help support or change their coping style to more of a problem/emotional coping style.

Cognitive Behavioural Therapy

Cognitive behavioral therapy (CBT) is a psycho-social intervention that seeks to improve mental health by challenging and changing unhelpful cognitive thoughts and behaviors, improving emotional regulation, and developing coping strategies [18]. Another CBT that significantly impacts illness management is adherence enhancement, which focuses on fostering a collaborative therapeutic alliance that allows the patient to discuss problems related to treatment adherence. The therapist then determines if such problems are practical (e.g., financial challenges, inadequate education) or psychological (e.g., inadequate motivation, overwhelming stress, inaccurate beliefs, family beliefs), and then helps patients develop strategies that are tailored to increase the likelihood of adherence [19].

While CBT has been proposed to help acne patients manage proper treatment behaviors, it has most widely been studied in psoriasis patients [20]. CBT, including one-on-one, group-based, and online programs, is probably the most widely studied treatment with clear evidence of a positive effect on psoriasis activity, distress, and quality of life, especially if therapy is tailored to the individual [21–25]. In the online program, patients listened to simulated patients talk about common experiences and completed short assignments on self-esteem, thinking styles, coping skills, depression, and stress [24]. While online-CBT improved physical functioning ($p = 0.03$) and impact on daily activities ($p = 0.04$) compared to control, it did not improve psychological functioning ($p = 0.32$), up to 6 months after treatment compared to baseline. However, these studies highlight the promise of therapist-guided, individually tailored CBT to improve physical functioning and reduce the impact of psoriasis on daily activities in patients with a psychological risk profile [25]. Establishing a good therapeutic relationship may be an important factor that influences treatment outcomes in CBT interventions.

Self-Management

Self-management is a patient's ability to manage symptoms, treatments, and physical and psychological consequences associated with a chronic condition. Since patients, not providers, are responsible for day-to-day disease management, patients must be more actively involved in their care through self-management. Evidence suggests that self-management interventions effectively increase patient knowledge, symptom management, and health status [26]. Self-management may help bridge the gap between patients' needs and the ability of healthcare to meet those needs.

There is increasing interest in developing self-management interventions for patients [27–29]. Educational interventions teach parents to better understand the need for medical interventions and effective disease management. The content of educational interventions may include disease information, treatment instructions, management and prevention strategies. Approaches include pamphlets, workshops, programs, online video education, and Web-based interventions [30–33]. However, interventions solely based on education are unlikely to bring about health behavior change [33]. Real health behavior change occurs when health education and self-efficacy are combined so that patients are more comfortable with self-management.

Self-Efficacy

Self-efficacy is the extent to which a person believes they are able to successfully initiate and complete actions needed to achieve a specific outcome [34]. Self-efficacy influences how individuals approach goals, tasks, and challenges. Individuals with high self-efficacy tend to confront challenging tasks, while individuals with low self-efficacy tend to avoid challenges altogether [34]. Interventions that strengthen patient self-efficacy result in positive changes in health behaviors and improved health outcomes [28, 35, 36]. There are four key sources of self-efficacy: mastery, vicarious experience, verbal persuasion, and emotional regulation.

This approach has been applied to adult psoriasis patients with promising results. The intervention consisted of four components based on the four sources of self-efficacy: a nurse-led group learning experience, supporting written and audio-visual material, a follow-up telephone consultation, and a relaxation resource. While intervention participants had a modest reduction in psoriasis severity, there was insufficient power to detect significance.

Interventions to evaluate and promote parental self-efficacy have been applied to atopic dermatitis [27–29]. One such intervention was an eczema educational program, which involved measuring parental self-efficacy both before and after the program. The eczema program intervention was based on the self-efficacy construct and consisted of a nurse-led session designed to generate group interaction, provide opportunities for shared learning, and offer mutual support [37]. The intervention enhanced the self-efficacy score of participants, meaning increased self-efficacy in managing eczema and symptoms [28]. A web-based education program similarly increased the self-efficacy of mothers [27]. Further research into self-efficacy may help researchers plan patient education programs, measure the impact of patient education programs, and detect individual differences in self-efficacy between patients.

Self-Awareness

Patients may have limited control in their behavior, emotions, and thoughts in the pursuit of long-term goals. Appropriate medication usage may lead to decreased time for other tasks, thus decreasing a patient's motivation for adherence. For example, a psoriasis patient may forgo using a topical medication because she has a social function and does not want the cream to show. Additionally, patients may have internal conflicts between prioritizing adhering to medication regimens with other responsibilities [38]. A mother may feel guilty spending time applying medication to her child with eczema and not spending time with her other children. Even if they are adhering to their medication, patients may still experience considerable distress, illness, and treatment uncertainty.

To aid self-regulation and promote adherence, patients are encouraged to reflect both on their beliefs about management of their illness and vital barriers that may be altering their adherence [39]. This approach may help patients identify potential solutions, help support psychological well-being, and enhance medication adherence. The identification and explicit recognition of potentially conflicting goals may itself be therapeutic and reduce distress. Increasing self-awareness of these conflicting goals may be therapeutic in itself by reducing expenditure of mental energy associated with internal conflict [40].

Patient Support Groups

There are many benefits to patient support groups. Support from peers may play a vital role in alleviating anxiety about the disease, improving health outcomes, and promoting medication adherence [41]. Studies demonstrate that peer support was associated with better outcomes among patients with chronic diseases [42]. Because psychological distress is frequently associated with skin disorders, support groups provide the social support, normalization of disease experience, and health literacy necessary to empower patients. Groups become valuable in normalizing a disease experience and conquering disease stigma, both of which have been found to cause nonadherence to medications in conditions such as psoriasis [38, 43]. In addition, increased health literacy through support groups help involve patients in the decision-making process for their disease management.

There is a growing trend to offer patient support programs to help patients and health care professionals better manage disease and optimize treatment. A study by the National Psoriasis Foundation found that patients in the US participating in patient support groups were more aware of treatment options, more likely to try more treatments, and were more satisfied with the treatment they were provided with [44]. Patient enrollment in the patient support group for those receiving treatment with adalimumab was associated with greater adherence, improved persistence, and reduced medical (all-cause and disease-related) and total health care costs [45].

Of course, the effectiveness of patient support groups depends on the content and support delivered at the sessions. A disparity in health literacy within various patient support groups has been noted and it has been suggested that coordinated efforts between organizations should be held to maximize the impact of patient group messaging [44]. Despite this, the empowerment that patients can get by being surrounded with others battling the same condition is a unique benefit all patient support groups can provide.

Physician-Centered Approaches

Because providers have such a significant role in adherence, designing interventions to influence their behaviour seems a reasonable strategy; however, few investigations on this subject have been reported in the literature. Physician-based strategies involve using motivational interviewing to help patients to better understand their behavior and its consequences, or helping learn by association, as discussed in the accountability section.

Motivational Interviewing

Motivational interviewing (MI) is a collaborative, patient-centered communications skill set that can increase behavior change by stimulating a patient's own internal motivation for change. Medical providers using MI can explore factors associated with medication nonadherence, assess patient ambivalence and/or resistance, and educate a patient to promote medication-adherent behaviors. Core components of MI include partnership (e.g. collaborative care), compassion (e.g. empathy, acknowledgement of people's thoughts/feelings), and evocation (e.g. eliciting patient-led solutions and management plans) [46]. The use of MI has expanded over the years from substance abuse to adherence to HIV-medications and more recently to adherence to other chronic medications [47]. Studies show that MI improves patients' adherence to medication, even with different exposure times, different modes (in-office or over the phone), and different counselors' background [48, 49].

MI has been explored in physicians treating psoriasis patients. A training program provided clinicians with MI skills to support behaviour change in patients with psoriasis and increase the clinicians' knowledge of psoriasis comorbidities. The training enhanced clinicians' ability to use MI skills to address behaviour change in the context of managing psoriasis and patient actors reported high levels of overall satisfaction with the consultation style used by clinicians following training. However, the clinicians' knowledge of psoriasis-related comorbidities did not increase after training, nor were they more likely to explain to patients how psoriasis and behavioural factors are associated. The researchers suggested this may have been because the training focused less on the relationships between psoriasis-associated conditions and behaviours, and more on how to address behaviour change with patients [50].

Another study evaluated the effects of a 3-month individual MI intervention in patients with psoriasis with the aim of inducing behaviour change in daily psoriasis treatment. The MI intervention had positive overall effects on disease severity, self-efficacy, psoriasis knowledge, and health behaviour change compared to the control group. The researchers suggested that the MI may have enhanced the patients' knowledge of psoriasis and reduced the risk of unhealthy lifestyle habits and nonadherence by encouraging healthy behaviours, facilitating the development of problem-solving skills, and providing emotional support and regular follow-up [51].

Addressing behavioural factors as part of psoriasis management is important because modification of lifestyle factors, medication adherence, and low mood can improve psoriasis outcomes and reduce the likelihood of developing or exacerbating psoriasis-related comorbidities. MI interventions to promote health behavior change can be tailored to individuals. MI can also change providers' approaches to discussions with their patients on psoriasis management. Moreover, MI can be carried out within the context of a consultation about psoriasis.

Accountability

The accountability derived from the expectation of a social interaction between the patient and the health care provider may affect patients' motivation to adhere to treatment. Accountability represents a potentially powerful tool to improve self-management, thereby promoting patients' adherence to treatment. Accountability refers to the implicit or explicit expectation that an individual may be called upon to account for his or her actions or inactions [52]. Accountability requires social presence—which can be by telephone, by email, or in person—the latter of which is considered the most influential [53–55].

In previous studies, adherence in psoriasis patients to topical treatment dropped from 85% at Week 1 to 51% at Week 8 ($p < 0.0001$) [56]. However, there were increases in adherence around the times of the Day 7, 14, 28, and 56 follow-up visits. These office visits may increase patient motivation to adhere to treatment by imparting a sense of accountability. Other studies have also shown that early follow-up visits can at least temporarily improve adherence [57–60].

Digital interactions have also improved patient adherence to treatment. In a study of acne patients, weekly contact via an Internet-based contest substantially improved adherence to treatment [53]. The acne study included 20 male and female participants, aged 13–18 years, with mild-to-moderate acne who were prescribed topical treatment for 12 weeks. Participants were randomized 1:1 to a control group or to an Internet-based survey group to receive weekly emails with a link to a survey to assess their acne severity and treatment. The median adherence rate was 74% in the digital-intervention group and 32% in the control group. These findings suggest that having patients report how they are doing may be an intervention for improving adherence [53].

System-Centered Approaches

In addition to patient-centered and physician-centered behavioural techniques, internal modifications to clinical practices can create a facilitative foundation for adherence interventions. The functioning of the health system influences patients' behavior in many ways. Systems direct providers' schedules, dictate appointment lengths, allocate resources, set fee structures, and establish organizational priorities. Interventions in the health system are higher order interventions affecting health policy, organization, financing of care, and quality of care programs. System-based approaches discussed in this chapter include scheduling longer appointment times, continuity of care, and communication with patients.

Longer Appointment Times

The World Health Organization (WHO) recommendations for systemic actions to increase adherence include increased appointment lengths to allow enough time to address adherence [61]. Having more time to build rapport with a patient and communicate the importance of adherence becomes therapeutically valuable in the long-run.

In one study, subjects with psoriasis exhibited a negative exponential relationship between the duration of clinic visits and adherence. In patients who had a clinic visit that lasted less than 3 minutes, only 8.8% of patients were adherent to the physician's recommendations. The percentage of adherent patients increased to 17.5% with a 3–5 minute visit, to 35.1% with a 5–10 minute visit, and to 28.1% with a visit lasting greater than 10 minutes [62]. Patients with a shorter visit were more likely to self-medicate, meaning they stopped using medications prescribed by doctors and instead sought other treatments. This suggested that good communication with doctors offered an important means to increase patients' adherence, which has been well documented [63].

Continuity of Care

WHO also recommends for increased continuity of care, such as being followed by the same physician, to increase proper adherence, presumably through increased physician-patient rapport and accountability [61]. However, it may not always be feasible for patients to see a single physician for the duration of their disease. For example, dermatologic conditions may be diagnosed by a dermatologist and referred to the patient's primary care provider for follow-up, or vice versa. In these cases, it may be useful to comment on the patient's pattern of adherence, or any specific strategies the patient found helpful in increasing adherence in the referral notes to keep the patient accountable.

Communication with Patient

Ongoing communication efforts, such as phone calls, emails, or messaging through a patient portal, keep the patient engaged in health care [62]. This strategy is simple and cost-effective for improving adherence [64]. Additionally, communication with patients serves as a reminder for the patient to take their medication [65]. Furthermore, this ongoing support may help patients build rapport and feel more comfortable with self-management. However, consistent involvement may be considered overly intrusive for some patients, which makes informed consent an integral part of such reminder systems [66].

Conclusion

Interventions to promote adherence are not consistently implemented in practice. Providers report lack of time, lack of knowledge, lack of incentives, and lack of feedback on performance as barriers. Clearly, nonadherence is not simply a problem experienced by patients. From the first visit to the follow-ups, providers can assess risks for nonadherence and deliver interventions to optimize adherence. To make this a reality, providers must have access to specific training in adherence management. Furthermore, health systems must design and support delivery systems that develop this training. Providers can learn to assess the potential for nonadherence, and then use this information to implement brief interventions to encourage and support progress towards adherence.

Adherence is a problem observed in patients, but it has roots beyond the patient. Nonadherence occurs in the context of treatment-related demands the patient must attempt to handle. These demands include learning new behaviours, altering daily routines, tolerating discomforts and inconveniences, and persisting in doing so while trying to function effectively in their various life-roles. While there is no behavioral magic bullet, there is substantial evidence identifying effective strategies for changing behavior.

Behavioral interventions to promote adherence may provide immediate, practical strategies to improve patient adherence and therefore treatment outcomes for patients suffering from chronic dermatological conditions. A common goal of behavioral interventions is to increase patients' involvement in care, thereby promoting better patient adherence. Improved self-efficacy and self-management enables patients may lead to better adherence, which leads to better health outcomes and reduced health care costs [67]. For dermatology patients to achieve fuller effects of medical therapies, providers need to better understand and more investigation into behavioral interventions to promote adherence.

Conflicts of Interest Dr. Steven R. Feldman is a speaker for Taro. He is a consultant and speaker for Galderma, Abbvie, Celgene, Abbott Labs, Lilly, Janssen, Novartis Pharmaceuticals and Leo Pharma Inc. Dr. Feldman has received grants from Galderma, Janssen, Abbott Labs, Abbvie, Celgene, Taro, Sanofi, Celgene, Novartis Pharmaceuticals, Qurient, Pfizer Inc. and Anacor. He is a consultant for Advance Medical, Caremark, Gerson Lehrman Group, Guidepoint Global, Kikaku, Lilly, Merck & Co Inc., Mylan, Pfizer Inc., Qurient, Sanofi, Sienna, Sun Pharma, Suncare Research, Valeant, and Xenoport. Dr. Feldman is the founder, chief technology officer and holds stock in Causa Research. Dr. Feldman holds stock and is majority owner in Medical Quality Enhancement Corporation. He receives Royalties from UpToDate, Informa and Xlibris.

Dr. Adrian Pona, Dr. Abigail Cline, Dr. Masicampo, Monica Shah, and Felicia Tai have no conflicts of interest to disclose.

References

1. Wright S. Patient satisfaction in the context of cancer care. Ir J Psychol. 1998;19(2–3):274–82.
2. Godding V, Kruth M, Jamart J. Joint consultation for high-risk asthmatic children and their families, with pediatrician and child psychiatrist as co-therapists: model and evaluation. Fam Process. 1997;36(3):265–80.
3. Miller TA, Dimatteo MR. Importance of family/social support and impact on adherence to diabetic therapy. Diabetes Metab Syndr Obes. 2013;6:421–6.
4. Cockburn J, Thompson SC, Marks R, Jolley D, Schofield P, Hill D. Behavioural dynamics of a clinical trial of sunscreens for reducing solar keratoses in Victoria, Australia. J Epidemiol Community Health. 1997;51(6):716–21.

5. Oxman AD, Thomson MA, Davis DA, Haynes RB. No magic bullets: a systematic review of 102 trials of interventions to improve professional practice. CMAJ. 1995;153(10):1423–31.
6. Smiddy MP, O'Connell R, Creedon SA. Systematic qualitative literature review of health care workers' compliance with hand hygiene guidelines. Am J Infect Control. 2015;43(3):269–74.
7. McAleer MA, Mason DL, Cunningham S, O'Shea SJ, McCormick PA, Stone C, et al. Alcohol misuse in patients with psoriasis: identification and relationship to disease severity and psychological distress. Br J Dermatol. 2011;164(6):1256–61.
8. Murota H, Takeuchi S, Sugaya M, Tanioka M, Onozuka D, Hagihara A, et al. Characterization of socioeconomic status of Japanese patients with atopic dermatitis showing poor medical adherence and reasons for drug discontinuation. J Dermatol Sci. 2015;79(3):279–87.
9. Neri L, Peris K, Longo C, Calvieri S, Frascione P, Parodi A, et al. Physician-patient communication and patient-reported outcomes in the actinic keratosis treatment adherence initiative (AK-TRAIN): a multicenter, prospective, real-life study of treatment satisfaction, quality of life and adherence to topical field-directed therapy for the treatment of actinic keratosis in Italy. J Eur Acad Dermatol Venereol. 2019;33(1):93–107.
10. Kazemi T, Sachsman SM, Wilhalme HM, Goh C. Isotretinoin therapy: a retrospective cohort analysis of completion rates and factors associated with nonadherence. J Am Acad Dermatol. 2018;79(3):571–3.
11. Craşovan DI, Sava FA. Translation, adaptation, and validation on Romanian population of COPE questionnaire for coping mechanisms analysis. Cogn Brain Behav. 2013;17(1):61–76.
12. Kasparian NA, McLoone JK, Butow PN. Psychological responses and coping strategies among patients with malignant melanoma: a systematic review of the literature coping strategies and patients with melanoma. Arch Dermatol. 2009;145(12):1415–27.
13. Kirby JS, Sisic M, Tan J. Exploring coping strategies for patients with hidradenitis suppurativa coping strategies for patients with hidradenitis suppurativa letters. JAMA Dermatol. 2016;152(10):1166–7.
14. Wahl A, Hanestad BR, Wiklund I, Moum T. Coping and quality of life in patients with psoriasis. Qual Life Res. 1999;8(5):427–33.
15. Fawzy FI, Cousins N, Fawzy NW, Kemeny ME, Elashoff R, Morton D. A structured psychiatric intervention for cancer patients. I. Changes over time in methods of coping and affective disturbance. Arch Gen Psychiatry. 1990;47(8):720–5.
16. Papava I, Oancea C, Enatescu VR, Bredicean AC, Dehelean L, Romosan RS, et al. The impact of coping on the somatic and mental status of patients with COPD: a cross-sectional study. Int J Chron Obstruct Pulmon Dis. 2016;11:1343–51.
17. Albai A, Sima A, Papava I, Roman D, Andor B, Gafencu M. Association between coping mechanisms and adherence to diabetes-related self-care activities: a cross-sectional study. Patient Prefer Adherence. 2017;11:1235–41.
18. Beck JS. Cognitive behavior therapy: basics and beyond: New York: Guilford Press; 2011.
19. Sudak DM. CBT in patients with chronic illness. Psychiatr News. 2017;52:1.
20. Jung J, Hwang EJ. Do patients with acne need cognitive behavioral therapy? An analysis of patient knowledge and behavior. Int J Dermatol. 2012;51(11):1319–24.
21. Zachariae R, Oster H, Bjerring P, Kragballe K. Effects of psychologic intervention on psoriasis: a preliminary report. J Am Acad Dermatol. 1996;34(6):1008–15.
22. Fortune DG, Richards HL, Kirby B, Bowcock S, Main CJ, Griffiths CE. A cognitive-behavioural symptom management programme as an adjunct in psoriasis therapy. Br J Dermatol. 2002;146(3):458–65.
23. Fortune DG, Richards HL, Kirby B, McElhone K, Main CJ, Griffiths CE. Successful treatment of psoriasis improves psoriasis-specific but not more general aspects of patients' well-being. Br J Dermatol. 2004;151(6):1219–26.
24. Bundy C, Pinder B, Bucci S, Reeves D, Griffiths CE, Tarrier N. A novel, web-based, psychological intervention for people with psoriasis: the electronic Targeted Intervention for Psoriasis (eTIPs) study. Br J Dermatol. 2013;169(2):329–36.
25. van Beugen S, Ferwerda M, Spillekom-van Koulil S, Smit JV, Zeeuwen-Franssen MEJ, Kroft EBM, et al. Tailored therapist-guided internet-based cognitive behavioral treatment for psoriasis: a randomized controlled trial. Psychother Psychosom. 2016;85(5):297–307.
26. Barlow J, Wright C, Sheasby J, Turner A, Hainsworth J. Self-management approaches for people with chronic conditions: a review. Patient Educ Couns. 2002;48(2):177–87.
27. Son HK, Lim J. The effect of a web-based education programme (WBEP) on disease severity, quality of life and mothers' self-efficacy in children with atopic dermatitis. J Adv Nurs. 2014;70(10):2326–38.
28. Ersser SJ, Farasat H, Jackson K, Gardiner E, Sheppard ZA, Cowdell F. Parental self-efficacy and the management of childhood atopic eczema: development and testing of a new clinical outcome measure. Br J Dermatol. 2015;173(6):1479–85.
29. Mitchell AE, Fraser JA. Parents' self-efficacy, outcome expectations, and self-reported task performance when managing atopic dermatitis in children: instrument reliability and validity. Int J Nurs Stud. 2011;48(2):215–26.
30. Armstrong AW, Kim RH, Idriss NZ, Larsen LN, Lio PA. Online video improves clinical outcomes in adults with atopic dermatitis: a randomized controlled trial. J Am Acad Dermatol. 2011;64(3):502–7.

31. Santer M, Muller I, Yardley L, Burgess H, Selinger H, Stuart BL, et al. Supporting self-care for families of children with eczema with a web-based intervention plus health care professional support: pilot randomized controlled trial. J Med Internet Res. 2014;16(3):e70.

32. van Os-Medendorp H, van Leent-de Wit I, de Bruin-Weller M, Knulst A. Usage and users of online self-management programs for adult patients with atopic dermatitis and food allergy: an explorative study. JMIR Res Protoc. 2015;4(2):e57.

33. Ersser SJ, Cowdell F, Latter S, Gardiner E, Flohr C, Thompson AR, et al. Psychological and educational interventions for atopic eczema in children. Cochrane Database Syst Rev. 2014;1:CD004054.

34. Bandura A. Self-efficacy: toward a unifying theory of behavioral change. Psychol Rev. 1977;84(2):191–215.

35. Lorig KR, Sobel DS, Stewart AL, Brown BW Jr, Bandura A, Ritter P, et al. Evidence suggesting that a chronic disease self-management program can improve health status while reducing hospitalization: a randomized trial. Med Care. 1999;37(1):5–14.

36. Ersser SJ, Cowdell FC, Nicholls PG, Latter SM, Healy E. A pilot randomized controlled trial to examine the feasibility and efficacy of an educational nursing intervention to improve self-management practices in patients with mild-moderate psoriasis. J Eur Acad Dermatol Venereol. 2011;26(6):738–45.

37. Jackson K, Ersser SJ, Dennis H, Farasat H, More A. The eczema education Programme: intervention development and model feasibility. J Eur Acad Dermatol Venereol. 2014;28(7):949–56.

38. Thorneloe RJ, Bundy C, Griffiths CEM, Ashcroft DM, Cordingley L. Nonadherence to psoriasis medication as an outcome of limited coping resources and conflicting goals: findings from a qualitative interview study with people with psoriasis. Br J Dermatol. 2017;176(3):667–76.

39. National Collaborating Centre for Primary C. National Institute for Health and Clinical Excellence: Guidance. Medicines adherence: involving patients in decisions about prescribed medicines and supporting adherence. London: Royal College of General Practitioners (UK); 2009.

40. Higginson S, Mansell W, Wood AM. An integrative mechanistic account of psychological distress, therapeutic change and recovery: the perceptual control theory approach. Clin Psychol Rev. 2011;31(2):249–59.

41. Penninx BWJH, Kriegsman DMW, van Eijk JTM, Boeke AJP, Deeg DJH. Differential effect of social support on the course of chronic disease: a criteria-based literature study. Fam Syst Health. 1996;14(2):223–44.

42. Chlebowy DO, Hood S, LaJoie AS. Facilitators and barriers to self-management of type 2 diabetes among urban African American adults: focus group findings. Diabetes Educ. 2010;36(6):897–905.

43. Thorneloe RJ, Bundy C, Griffiths CE, Ashcroft DM, Cordingley L. Adherence to medication in patients with psoriasis: a systematic literature review. Br J Dermatol. 2013;168(1):20–31.

44. Eissing L, Radtke MA, Zander N, Augustin M. Barriers to guideline-compliant psoriasis care: analyses and concepts. J Eur Acad Dermatol Venereol. 2016;30(4):569–75.

45. Rubin DT, Mittal M, Davis M, Johnson S, Chao J, Skup M. Impact of a patient support program on patient adherence to adalimumab and direct medical costs in Crohn's disease, ulcerative colitis, rheumatoid arthritis, psoriasis, psoriatic arthritis, and ankylosing spondylitis. J Manag Care Spec Pharm. 2017;23(8):859–67.

46. Miller WR, Rollnick S. Motivational interviewing: helping people change: New York: Guilford Press; 2012.

47. Zomahoun HTV, Guenette L, Gregoire JP, Lauzier S, Lawani AM, Ferdynus C, et al. Effectiveness of motivational interviewing interventions on medication adherence in adults with chronic diseases: a systematic review and meta-analysis. Int J Epidemiol. 2017;46(2):589–602.

48. Palacio A, Garay D, Langer B, Taylor J, Wood BA, Tamariz L. Motivational interviewing improves medication adherence: a systematic review and meta-analysis. J Gen Intern Med. 2016;31(8):929–40.

49. Teeter BS, Kavookjian J. Telephone-based motivational interviewing for medication adherence: a systematic review. Transl Behav Med. 2014;4(4):372–81.

50. Chisholm A, Nelson PA, Pearce CJ, Littlewood AJ, Kane K, Henry AL, et al. Motivational interviewing-based training enhances clinicians' skills and knowledge in psoriasis: findings from the Pso Well® study. Br J Dermatol. 2017;176(3):677–86.

51. Larsen MH, Krogstad AL, Aas E, Moum T, Wahl AK. A telephone-based motivational interviewing intervention has positive effects on psoriasis severity and self-management: a randomized controlled trial. Br J Dermatol. 2014;171(6):1458–69.

52. Lerner JS, Tetlock PE. Accounting for the effects of accountability. Psychol Bull. 1999;125(2):255–75.

53. Yentzer BA, Wood AA, Sagransky MJ, O'Neill JL, Clark AR, Williams LL, et al. An internet-based survey and improvement of acne treatment outcomes. Arch Dermatol. 2011;147(10):1223–4.

54. Davis SA, Lin HC, Yu CH, Balkrishnan R, Feldman SR. Underuse of early follow-up visits: a missed opportunity to improve patients' adherence. J Drugs Dermatol. 2014;13(7):833–6.

55. Laffer MS, Feldman SR. Improving medication adherence through technology: analyzing the managing meds video challenge. Skin Res Technol. 2014;20(1):62–6.

56. Carroll CL, Feldman SR, Camacho FT, Manuel JC, Balkrishnan R. Adherence to topical therapy decreases during the course of an 8-week psoriasis clinical trial: commonly used methods of measuring adherence to topical therapy overestimate actual use. J Am Acad Dermatol. 2004;51(2):212–6.
57. Shah A, Yentzer BA, Feldman SR. Timing of return office visit affects adherence to topical treatment in patients with atopic dermatitis: an analysis of 5 studies. Cutis. 2013;91(2):105–7.
58. Sagransky MJ, Yentzer BA, Williams LL, Clark AR, Taylor SL, Feldman SR. A randomized controlled pilot study of the effects of an extra office visit on adherence and outcomes in atopic dermatitis. Arch Dermatol (United States). 2010;146:1428–30.
59. Feldman SR, Camacho FT, Krejci-Manwaring J, Carroll CL, Balkrishnan R. Adherence to topical therapy increases around the time of office visits. J Am Acad Dermatol. 2007;57(1):81–3.
60. Yentzer BA, Gosnell AL, Clark AR, Pearce DJ, Balkrishnan R, Camacho FT, et al. A randomized controlled pilot study of strategies to increase adherence in teenagers with acne vulgaris. J Am Acad Dermatol. 2011;64(4):793–5.
61. Sabate E, Sabaté E, Organisation mondiale de la s, World Health O, Unaids. Adherence to long-term therapies: evidence for action. New York: World Health Organization; 2003.
62. Zhang L, Yang H, Wang Y, Chen Y, Zhou H, Shen Z. Self-medication of psoriasis in southwestern China. Dermatology (Basel, Switzerland). 2014;228(4):368–74.
63. Richards HL, Fortune DG, Griffiths CE. Adherence to treatment in patients with psoriasis. J Eur Acad Dermatol Venereol. 2006;20(4):370–9.
64. Fenerty SD, West C, Davis SA, Kaplan SG, Feldman SR. The effect of reminder systems on patients' adherence to treatment. Patient Prefer Adherence. 2012;6:127–35.
65. Yelamos O, Ros S, Puig L. Improving patient outcomes in psoriasis: strategies to ensure treatment adherence. Psoriasis (Auckland, NZ). 2015;5:109–15.
66. Feldman SR, Vrijens B, Gieler U, Piaserico S, Puig L, van de Kerkhof P. Treatment adherence intervention studies in dermatology and guidance on how to support adherence. Am J Clin Dermatol. 2017;18(2):253–71.
67. Horwitz RI, Horwitz SM. Adherence to treatment and health outcomes. Arch Intern Med. 1993;153(16):1863–8.

Chapter 5
Adherence in Pediatric Populations

Abigail Cline, Adrian Pona, and Steven R. Feldman

Introduction

Upwards of 50% of pediatric patients with chronic health conditions are considered to be nonadherent to medical treatment regimens. As such, improving self-management and adherence are paramount to not only improving health outcomes, but pediatric adjustment to chronic disease. Dermatologic conditions in pediatric populations put children at an increased risk for low self-esteem, depression, anxiety, social isolation, and suicidal ideation [1]. Social reactions to cutaneous disease are more devastating to pediatric populations, and appearance-related concerns are one of the dominant experiences of adolescents [2]. The impact of skin conditions on a pediatric patients' quality of life warrant early recognition and treatment to decrease their risk of physical and psychologic morbidity.

Treatment adherence is particularly challenging in pediatric populations because of family dynamics and functioning, caregiver and child characteristics, and child health outcomes. When patients are young, caregivers are often responsible for medication administration, but this responsibility shifts to the patients as they mature. This shift can complicate treatment adherence. Furthermore, both caregivers and providers should emphasize the importance of adherence in young patients to instill a sense of self-management that can persist into adulthood. Poor adherence results in poor health outcomes, which can lead to misconceptions about treatment efficacy, sometimes creating what appears to be "treatment-resistant" disease.

Promoting acceptable levels of adherence requires examining parent and child variables that facilitate or impede adherence to treatment recommendations. This chapter aims to explore the complexity of adherence in pediatric dermatology patients. We discuss barriers to adherence for the pediatric population followed by approaches that can be used to address adherence issues.

A. Cline (✉) · A. Pona
Department of Dermatology, Wake Forest School of Medicine, Winston-Salem, NC, USA
e-mail: aecline@wakehealth.edu

S. R. Feldman
Departments of Dermatology, Pathology and Social Sciences & Health Policy, Wake Forest School of Medicine, Winston-Salem, NC, USA

© Springer Nature Switzerland AG 2020   41
S. R. Feldman et al. (eds.), *Treatment Adherence in Dermatology*, Updates in Clinical Dermatology,
https://doi.org/10.1007/978-3-030-27809-0_5

Common Barriers to Adherence in Pediatric Populations

Caregivers and pediatric patients have common and unique factors that affect adherence (Table 5.1). Shared barriers include treatment factors, medication cost, and treatment expectations [3]. Treatment factors include medication tolerability, regimen complexity, and cost. Vehicle preference and selection of treatment in pediatrics may be difficult if the patient and caregiver have differing preferences. In younger pediatric patients, treatments will likely be chosen by the caregiver who administers the medication. In older teenagers, treatments may be chosen by the patient or the caregiver. Decisional discord may lead to low adherence, especially if either party is not in full agreement of the treatment plan [4, 5].

Studies have demonstrated that parents with greater resources exhibit better adherence than parents with fewer resources [6]. Pediatric patients also rely on their caregiver to purchase the medication. When caregivers of pediatric dermatology patients were surveyed about factors leading to nonadherence, cost of medicine was among the most important reasons [7]. Strategies to lower medication cost include creating more cost effective treatment plans, and using generic medications when possible.

Caregiver and patient expectations set the course for treatment. For example, treatment outcomes for dermatological conditions typically occur gradually. If caregivers and patients are uninformed about the likelihood of gradual outcomes and expect full and early clearance, they may become frustrated and less adherent. Caregivers and patients also may not believe the condition as chronic, thereby requiring continuous therapy. For example, caregivers and patients may have little understanding of the maintenance role of emollients in preventing atopic dermatitis flare-ups.

Additionally, behavioral issues of patients and caregivers can undermine adherence and treatment outcomes. Children with chronic health problems are at increased risk of behavioral and emotional difficulties [8, 9]. Mood disorders, such as depression, may interfere with patient adherence because of poor concentration, fatigue, loss of interest in activities, sleep/ appetite disruption, and irritable mood [10]. Similarly, caregiver depression can hinder parental engagement in following the regimen [11]. Child behavior problems are associated with greater parent-reported difficulties with illness management [12]. Caregivers may also feel the time spent applying treatments on one child impacts the time and energy to expend on siblings and partners. If a child is resistant to receiving treatment, caregivers often pay the cost with their own emotional well-being [13].

Table 5.1 Barriers to treatment adherence in pediatric patients/caregivers

Treatment factors
Complicated treatment regimen
Poor tolerability of treatment (e.g. treatment too messy, greasy)
Time-consuming treatment regimen
Medication cost
Common factors between caregiver and patient
Delayed treatment outcomes
Mental health disorders/behavioral issues
Caregiver/parent factors
Poor communication
Fear of medication side effects (corticosteroid phobia)
Patient factors
Age-related and developmental stage-related limitations
Difficulty with transfer of treatment responsibility during adolescence

Caregiver-Centered Barriers

Pediatric patients often rely on their parent or guardian to promote treatment adherence through the purchase and/or actual administration of medications. About 47.8% of prescriptions for children attending a dermatology outpatient clinic remained unfilled [14]. Even when medications were directly supplied to parents and regular follow-ups were provided, adherence rates were as low as 32% [15]. Pediatric patients also depend on a parent or guardian to be in attendance to consent for procedures and assist with transportation. Scheduling conflicts between caregiver and child can interfere with adherence to treatments that require frequent visits, such as phototherapy.

Caregiver concern about side effects is also a major factor in nonadherence [7]. The fear of adverse effects of topical corticosteroids is called "steroid phobia" [16]. Steroid phobia is increasingly recognized as playing a key role in poor treatment adherence, which leads to poor treatment outcomes and disease flares. Originally used to describe an irrational fear of corticosteroids, steroid phobia has been broadened to include the vague negative feelings and beliefs about using topical corticosteroids [17]. As many as 80.7% of patients reported having fears about topical corticosteroids, and 36% admitted to treatment nonadherence due to concern about steroid-related adverse effects [16]. Steroid phobia correlates with several factors, including the belief that topical corticosteroid agents pass through the skin into the bloodstream, a lack of trust in the health care provider, and discrepancies in the education about their use. Common concerns about topical corticosteroids include skin thinning, the potential of topical corticosteroids to affect growth and development, and nonspecific long-term effects. This fear can further complicate treatment as patients often initially depend on their caregivers to administer medications.

Child-Centered Barriers

Barriers to adherence that are unique to children include instructional compliance and developmental level. Children may not be aware that they have a problem, or they may not be motivated to work on it. For example, the management of atopic dermatitis is a complex process with multiple steps that have to be followed by the child. These include disrupting current activity, undressing, bathing, and receiving topical applications that may feel uncomfortable. Children are not naturally motivated to follow such complex instructions and may therefore resist implementing a treatment routine. Maintaining a treatment regimen requires the child to be under good instructional control or the child will often not comply with the program.

Developmental level also influences treatment adherence, especially when treatments require the child to actively participate. Caregivers are often responsible for medication adherence in young children, whereas adherence for older children or adolescents becomes a process of shared responsibility. Adolescence is a critical period for many children with a chronic medical condition. Adolescents often fare worse with regimen adherence than younger children across multiple pediatric conditions [18–20]. With adolescence also comes increasing general responsibility, and many caregivers and providers transition treatment responsibility to the adolescent. This transition can lead to an increase in caregiver–child conflict over treatment management and adherence [21]. Specifically, as children move into adolescence, they begin taking control of their bodies and may want more responsibility in decision making. Despite this desire for more responsibility, adolescents may need more support from caregivers and medical providers in developing and following their treatment regimens.

Table 5.2 Adherence
assessment

| **Time constraints** |
| Identify priorities and enhance time management |
| **Financial resources** |
| Prescribe generic, affordable options |
| Work with pharmacy or insurance company on financial assistance |
| **Forgetfulness** |
| Set reminds (alarms, texts), frequent follow-up |
| **Regimen complexity** |
| Simplify regimen with combination treatments |
| **Prior treatments** |
| Discuss problems with prior treatment options and regimens |
| **Mental health/family issues** |
| Acknowledge, assess, normalize, and validate |
| Involve psychologist if necessary |

Adherence Assessment

Nonadherence can occur even with the most committed families. Providers can perform a functional assessment to identify barriers to treatment adherence specific to patients and caregivers (Table 5.2). Providers may find it helpful to ask families about nonadherent behaviors, antecedents that trigger nonadherence, and factors that contribute to nonadherence (i.e., time constraints, medication cost, forgetfulness, regimen complexity). If families are unable to identify barriers, discussing their prior treatment experiences may highlight potential barriers. If treatments are recommended for specific daytime or nighttime routines, providers should discuss potential problem-solving interventions. For example, reviewing a patient's typical bedtime routine can help families think more clearly about integrating recommended treatments. Identifying reasons for nonadherence in patients and caregivers can help providers develop treatment plans that are ultimately employed with greater adherence.

During these discussions, providers should also screen for psychosocial factors and stress associated with pediatric dermatologic disorders, including the important role of mental health. Challenges facing caregivers of children with chronic health conditions include competently and consistently implementing a treatment regimen to which the child may be uncooperative or resistant [22]. Addressing mental health issues or problematic family functioning and communication may be necessary for optimizing adherence. Families can also be referred for psychological care when family communication strategies limit the ability to effectively share treatment responsibilities, especially among adolescents, or when parental mental health issues (eg, depression) impede treatment management.

If the patient and caregivers feel that their concerns to the successful implementation of the medical regimen have not been addressed, then they will likely be less successful in adhering [23]. Medical providers should ensure that caregivers and patient understand the logistics of completing their medical regimen and that following the medical regimen will lead to improved health outcomes.

Approaches and Techniques to Facilitate Treatment Adherence

Setting the stage for enhancing treatment adherence with children and adolescents generally involves attending three broad areas: (a) relationship building and support, (b) education, and (c) skills training and motivation. Meta-analyses of treatment adherence suggested that when interventions use more than one strategy for improving adherence, they are more effective [24–26].

Table 5.3 Relationship building and support

Patient rapport
Build a relationship with the caregiver and the patient to boost cooperation
"Normalize" the problem with children/adolescents and provide anecdotes
Treatment preference
Ask both caregiver and patient about individual preference
Try to find a compromise
Confidence assessment
Give 1–10 scale about confidence using treatment and adhering to treatment
Provide positive reinforcement/problem-solve barriers
Early follow-up
Phone call, email, or return visit
Ask about nonadherence and treatment difficulties

Relationship Building and Support

The first step to improving adherence is to build a foundation that fosters trust and accountability between the provider, the patient, and the caregiver (Table 5.3). The caregiver may ultimately decide treatment and can potentially serve as a strong motivating factor for adherence and the development of self-management skills. Thus, building a rapport with young children may not be an integral part of promoting adherence. However, in situations where the child is responsible for a particular component of treatment (e.g., submitting to phototherapy or topical applications), the provider should focus on building rapport with the child to boost cooperation with treatment. Because adolescents are more actively involved in medical treatments, establishing rapport with adolescents can increase their treatment adherence. With young children and adolescents, providers should "normalize" the problem by telling patients that many children/adolescents with similar dermatological issues improved with the recommended treatment. This is an example of using anecdotal evidence to increase patient adherence.

Listening to caregiver and patient preference further strengthen the provider-patient relationship. Caregivers and patients may be more likely to adhere to a medicine they have selected rather than one that is selected for them. Caregivers and patients often find frustration with topical medication application to be a significant barrier to adherence. Therefore, providers should discuss a range of possible topical medications and when to apply the topical medication to minimize this negative experience. Families may need time to work together to decide on potential treatment options to ensure it is tailored and feasible for the patient. Studies outside of dermatology show that when parents approve of treatment and feel it is working, pediatric patients have higher adherence rates [5].

With barriers identified and a plan to address these barriers in place, providers can assess caregiver/parent confidence with following the treatment regimen, feasibly using a 1–10 scale. For example, assessing confidence levels can highlight a caregiver's strengths ("You rate your confidence at a 7; what helps you feel that confident?"). At the same time, rating can help enhance motivation for increased adherence ("You rate your confidence at a 7; what would it take for you to be at an 8?") [27]. If there are barriers that cannot be addressed by the medical provider or the current medical regimen, options include switching treatment plans to one with fewer barriers or referring to a psychologist to provide a more detailed assessment of adherence issues.

As new treatment behaviors are developing, follow-up within 2 to 4 weeks can promote adherence by offering the chance for reinstruction or barrier mitigation [28]. This can be done either through contacting the patient or early follow-up visits. While contact is often done via phone calls and follow-up visits, email and electronic medical record patient portals is inexpensive and convenient. Having an early follow-up visits to check on how well the medication is working holds patients and caregivers accountable to use the medication. The accountability inherent in the social interaction between a patient and a healthcare professional affects patients' motivation to adhere to treatment. This leads to improved initial adherence and short-term outcomes, which helps secure good long-term adherence. Whether through contact or follow-up visits, providers should inquire about the treatment regimen, assess adherence, and express approval for caregivers/patients following the treatment regimen correctly. Providers should acknowledge there are likely to be some adherence challenges and maintain a constructive solution-focused approach.

Treatment Education Interventions

The more knowledge caregivers have about disease, the better their motivation and adherence to disease management will be. Education interventions for atopic dermatitis have been developing over the past decade. Education interventions for other chronic medical conditions, such as asthma, are based on the idea that education limited to handouts and brief explanations may not be sufficient [29]. Education interventions are especially applicable for those with severe disease, diminished quality of life, and lack of therapeutic adherence. Studies have empirically shown that improved self-management interventions increase child and caregiver quality of life [30–34].

Educational programs for caregivers of children with chronic dermatological conditions contribute towards comprehensive, family-oriented management [35]. Educational interventions aim to enable patients and caregivers to solve problems arising from chronic diseases at home. Treatment education allows for explanations and discussions of the dermatological condition and appropriate treatments (Table 5.4) [26]. Educating patients and families on disease pathophysiology and likely clinical course can enhance treatment motivation and link treatment options directly to the cause. Using developmentally appropriate language is important so that children and adolescents of all ages can understand their condition and treatment regimen. Caregiver training reduced the severity of atopic dermatitis considerably, suggesting caregiver education is an important factor in achieving a positive long-term outcome [36–38].

Education interventions can also help dissuade caregiver concerns about adverse effects, such as steroid phobia. Caregivers worried about possible side effects of topical steroids may benefit from additional education about appropriate times to start and stop topical steroid therapy. Patients who feel that their provider is following them closely for potential adverse effects may also feel more comfortable with topical corticosteroid use [39].

Providing additional ways for patients and parents to remember and become familiar with the treatment plan may further increase adherence. In addition to directly educating patients and families, providers should give a detailed, simple written action plan. The pediatric atopic dermatitis literature

Table 5.4 Treatment education

Medical knowledge
Discuss pathophysiology, severity, contributing factors, and clinical course
Treatment options
Discuss therapies and link them to the pathophysiology of the disease
Discuss efficacy, safety concerns, and potential side effects
Establish patient expectations for improvement
Side effects
Give additional education about potential adverse effects to worried caregivers
Written action plans
Define type of intervention, medication, frequency, and location
Provide adjustments during flare/maintenance
Consider color-coding system

demonstrates the utility of clear, direct written action plans [26, 40, 41]. Written action plans include a clear outline of the medical regimen including the type of task (e.g., bathing, application of topical medications, and dosing of oral medications), the frequency and location of the application of the medications, and how to adjust the intensity of treatments when symptoms are better/worse. In particular, families benefit from a clear definition of what constitutes a "flare" and how to adjust specific treatments. Some written action plans used a stoplight color-coding system to aid in health literacy and understanding of complicated medical regimen associated with atopic dermatitis [42].

Written action plans help parents determine when an immediate physician visit is needed, which cuts down on unnecessary visits and avoids harmful delays when physician care is needed. Written action plans may also provide a simple daily reminder to apply medications. Finally, written action plans provide a communication aid for healthcare providers and parents. This feature may improve parents' understanding of treatment goals, and thus their motivation to adhere to treatment regimens.

Motivation Interventions

Skill and motivation significantly influence caregiver and patient adherence. Some patients may lack the skills to implement a treatment protocol, whereas others have sufficient skill but lack motivation. While skill deficits can be overcome with educational interventions and written action plans, motivation deficits rely on psychological approaches (Table 5.5). A number of interconnected factors affecting the caregiver's and child's motivation can influence adherence to a treatment regimen. Common factors include the amount of time and effort the treatment requires, the degree to which the treatment interferes with other activities, and the ongoing results of the treatment. General strategies for improving motivation include simplifying the treatment regimen, establishing a reward system favoring adherence, and positive reinforcement.

The goal of simplifying treatment is typically to modify treatments so that they are less complex, require less effort, and involve less disruption to typical child and family schedules. An easier treatment regimen reduces the burden of treatment and increases the likelihood that parents and caregivers will adhere. Providers should attempt to prescribe low-cost and fast-acting medications as parents are more likely to pick up prescriptions they can afford. Furthermore, providers can provide instructions that allow pharmacists to offer a similar but less expensive treatment option if available. If slow-acting agents are necessary, providers can consider pairing them with fast-acting so that patients can still see rapid improvement. Multiple prescriptions complicate regimens and increase the chance patients will not correctly follow treatment [43]. Prescribing a single product that contains two more medications reduces the burden of treatment and increase adherence [44].

Age-appropriate methods of improving motivation and therefore adherence are valuable when treating children. Rewards, such as token economics and sticker charts, can improve adherence. Token economics involve a reward system in which children are provided with tokens or points for engaging in desirable behaviors. The tokens can then be exchanged for preferred items and activities that parents are willing to supply. Positive reinforcement techniques such as sticker charts may also increase motivation to adhere to treatment regimens. Receiving a sticker for each medication application gives

Table 5.5 Motivation interventions

Simplifying treatment regimen
Prescribe low-cost, fast-acting, medications
Consider combination therapies and once daily dosing
Positive reinforcement
Token economics, sticker charts
Gradually shape behavior for better autonomy

children an immediate sense of accomplishment and helps remind caregivers whether a treatment was completed and when a new dose is due [3, 45]. In several studies, sticker charts improved adherence and this effect was maintained for months after the initial intervention. Better adherence correlated with better clinical outcomes in some, but not all, studies. The majority of the participants in these studies were aged 3 to 12, a population highly receptive to operant conditioning interventions [45].

Positive reinforcement interventions in children with chronic disease improve adherence and clinical outcomes [46]. Operant conditioning theory describes positive reinforcement as pairing a desired behavior with a positive event, and increasing the likelihood of that behavior to occur again. An effective form of operant conditioning involves shaping, whereby behaviors required to achieve the same reward become increasingly difficult or the reward is increasingly diminished. In this manner, subjects are less dependent on the immediate reward and learn to produce the behavior autonomously [47].

Conclusion

Treatment outcomes depend on treatment adherence. Providers can maximize adherence by identifying barriers to adherence, educating patients and caregivers on disease and treatments, ensuring that treatment regimens are affordable and appropriate for patient/caregiver skill level, providing detailed written action plans, and following-up with patients about their treatment course. When medical treatment is shared by family members, success relies on an understanding of treatment responsibilities. If treatment responsibilities are not understood or discussed within the family, treatment adherence and management suffers. While interventions can be implemented for patients or caregiver factors independently, intervening with both caregivers and patients is ideal. We have attempted to show that adherence is multifactorial, and how to manipulate a broad range of variables to promote it. Although none of these variables guarantees full adherence, they do improve the chances that patients and caregivers will engage in sufficient adherence to increase the probability of a positive outcome.

Funding sources None

Conflicts of Interest Dr. Feldman is a speaker for Taro. He is a consultant and speaker for Galderma, Abbvie, Celgene, Abbott Labs, Lilly, Janssen, Novartis Pharmaceuticals and Leo Pharma Inc. Dr. Feldman has received grants from Galderma, Janssen, Abbott Labs, Abbvie, Celgene, Taro, Sanofi, Celgene, Novartis Pharmaceuticals, Qurient, Pfizer Inc. and Anacor. He is a consultant for Advance Medical, Caremark, Gerson Lehrman Group, Guidepoint Global, Kikaku, Lilly, Merck & Co Inc., Mylan, Pfizer Inc., Qurient, Sanofi, Sienna, Sun Pharma, Suncare Research, Valeant, and Xenoport. Dr. Feldman is the founder, chief technology officer and holds stock in Causa Research. Dr. Feldman holds stock and is majority owner in Medical Quality Enhancement Corporation. He receives Royalties from UpToDate, Informa and Xlibris.

Abigail Cline and Adrian Pona have no conflicts of interest to disclose.

References

1. Gieler U, Gieler T, Kupfer JP. Acne and quality of life – impact and management. J Eur Acad Dermatol Venereol. 2015;29(S4):12–4.
2. Levenson J. Psychiatric issues in dermatology, Part 1: atopic dermatitis and psoriasis. Primary Psychiatry. 2008;15(7):35–8.
3. Ou HT, Feldman SR, Balkrishnan R. Understanding and improving treatment adherence in pediatric patients. Semin Cutan Med Surg. 2010;29(2):137–40.
4. Sisk BA, DuBois J, Kodish E, Wolfe J, Feudtner C. Navigating decisional discord: the pediatrician's role when child and parents disagree. Pediatrics. 2017;139(6):e20170234.

5. Nagae M, Nakane H, Honda S, Ozawa H, Hanada H. Factors affecting medication adherence in children receiving outpatient pharmacotherapy and parental adherence. J Child Adolesc Psychiatr Nurs. 2015;28(2):109–17.
6. Gong T, Lundholm C, Rejno G, Mood C, Langstrom N, Almqvist C. Parental socioeconomic status, childhood asthma and medication use–a population-based study. PLoS One. 2014;9(9):e106579.
7. Ellis RM, Koch LH, McGuire E, Williams JV. Potential barriers to adherence in pediatric dermatology. Pediatr Dermatol. 2011;28(3):242–4.
8. Blackman JA, Gurka MJ, Gurka KK, Oliver MN. Emotional, developmental and behavioural co-morbidities of children with chronic health conditions. J Paediatr Child Health. 2011;47(10):742–7.
9. Pinquart M, Shen Y. Behavior problems in children and adolescents with chronic physical illness: a meta-analysis. J Pediatr Psychol. 2011;36(9):1003–16.
10. DiMatteo MR, Lepper HS, Croghan TW. Depression is a risk factor for noncompliance with medical treatment: meta-analysis of the effects of anxiety and depression on patient adherence. Arch Intern Med. 2000;160(14):2101–7.
11. Cameron LD, Young MJ, Wiebe DJ. Maternal trait anxiety and diabetes control in adolescents with type 1 diabetes. J Pediatr Psychol. 2007;32(7):733–44.
12. Mitchell AE, Fraser JA, Ramsbotham J, Morawska A, Yates P. Childhood atopic dermatitis: a cross-sectional study of relationships between child and parent factors, atopic dermatitis management, and disease severity. Int J Nurs Stud. 2015;52(1):216–28.
13. Santer M, Burgess H, Yardley L, Ersser SJ, Lewis-Jones S, Muller I, et al. Managing childhood eczema: qualitative study exploring carers' experiences of barriers and facilitators to treatment adherence. J Adv Nurs. 2013;69(11):2493–501.
14. Storm A, Andersen SE, Benfeldt E, Serup J. One in 3 prescriptions are never redeemed: primary nonadherence in an outpatient clinic. J Am Acad Dermatol. 2008;59(1):27–33.
15. Krejci-Manwaring J, Tusa MG, Carroll C, Camacho F, Kaur M, Carr D, et al. Stealth monitoring of adherence to topical medication: adherence is very poor in children with atopic dermatitis. J Am Acad Dermatol. 2007;56(2):211–6.
16. Aubert-Wastiaux H, Moret L, Le Rhun A, Fontenoy AM, Nguyen JM, Leux C, et al. Topical corticosteroid phobia in atopic dermatitis: a study of its nature, origins and frequency. Br J Dermatol. 2011;165(4):808–14.
17. Charman CR, Morris AD, Williams HC. Topical corticosteroid phobia in patients with atopic eczema. Br J Dermatol. 2000;142(5):931–6.
18. Anderson BJ, Brackett J, Ho J, Laffel LM. An office-based intervention to maintain parent-adolescent teamwork in diabetes management. Impact on parent involvement, family conflict, and subsequent glycemic control. Diabetes Care. 1999;22(5):713–21.
19. Feinstein S, Keich R, Becker-Cohen R, Rinat C, Schwartz SB, Frishberg Y. Is noncompliance among adolescent renal transplant recipients inevitable? Pediatrics. 2005;115(4):969–73.
20. Masterson TL, Wildman BG, Newberry BH, Omlor GJ. Impact of age and gender on adherence to infection control guidelines and medical regimens in cystic fibrosis. Pediatr Pulmonol. 2011;46(3):295–301.
21. Hilliard ME, Guilfoyle SM, Dolan LM, Hood KK. Prediction of adolescents' glycemic control 1 year after diabetes-specific family conflict: the mediating role of blood glucose monitoring adherence. Arch Pediatr Adolesc Med. 2011;165(7):624–9.
22. Morawska A, Calam R, Fraser J. Parenting interventions for childhood chronic illness: a review and recommendations for intervention design and delivery. J Child Health Care. 2014;19(1):5–17.
23. Dabade TS, Feldman SR. We must think outside the box to understand nonadherence. Pediatr Dermatol. 2011;28(3):353.
24. Roter DL, Hall JA, Merisca R, Nordstrom B, Cretin D, Svarstad B. Effectiveness of interventions to improve patient compliance: a meta-analysis. Med Care. 1998;36(8):1138–61.
25. Kahana S, Drotar D, Frazier T. Meta-analysis of psychological interventions to promote adherence to treatment in pediatric chronic health conditions. J Pediatr Psychol. 2008;33(6):590–611.
26. Ersser SJ, Cowdell F, Latter S, Gardiner E, Flohr C, Thompson AR, et al. Psychological and educational interventions for atopic eczema in children. Cochrane Database Syst Rev. 2014;1:CD004054.
27. Shah KN, Cortina S, Ernst MM, Kichler JC. Psoriasis in childhood: effective strategies to improve treatment adherence. Psoriasis (Auckland, NZ). 2015;5:43–54.
28. Shah A, Yentzer BA, Feldman SR. Timing of return office visit affects adherence to topical treatment in patients with atopic dermatitis: an analysis of 5 studies. Cutis. 2013;91(2):105–7.
29. Barbarot S, Bernier C, Deleuran M, De Raeve L, Eichenfield L, El Hachem M, et al. Therapeutic patient education in children with atopic dermatitis: position paper on objectives and recommendations. Pediatr Dermatol. 2013;30(2):199–206.
30. Schuttelaar MLA, Vermeulen KM, Drukker N, Coenraads PJ. A randomized controlled trial in children with eczema: nurse practitioner vs. dermatologist. Br J Dermatol. 2009;162(1):162–70.
31. Chinn DJ, Poyner T, Sibley G. Randomized controlled trial of a single dermatology nurse consultation in primary care on the quality of life of children with atopic eczema. Br J Dermatol. 2002;146(3):432–9.

32. Grillo M, Gassner L, Marshman G, Dunn S, Hudson P. Pediatric atopic eczema: the impact of an educational intervention. Pediatr Dermatol. 2006;23(5):428–36.

33. Staab D, Diepgen TL, Fartasch M, Kupfer J, Lob-Corzilius T, Ring J, et al. Age related, structured educational programmes for the management of atopic dermatitis in children and adolescents: multicentre, randomised controlled trial. BMJ (Clinical Research Ed). 2006;332(7547):933–8.

34. Weber BM, Fontes Neto Pde T, Prati C, Soirefman M, Mazzotti NG, Barzenski B, et al. Improvement of pruritus and quality of life of children with atopic dermatitis and their families after joining support groups. J Eur Acad Dermatol Venereol. 2008;22(8):992–7.

35. Staab D, Von Rueden U, Kehrt R, Erhart M, Wenninger K, Kamtsiuris P, et al. Evaluation of a parental training program for the management of childhood atopic dermatitis. Pediatr Allergy Immunol. 2002;13(2):84–90.

36. Cork MJ, Britton J, Butler L, Young S, Murphy R, Keohane SG. Comparison of parent knowledge, therapy utilization and severity of atopic eczema before and after explanation and demonstration of topical therapies by a specialist dermatology nurse. Br J Dermatol. 2003;149(3):582–9.

37. Futamura M, Masuko I, Hayashi K, Ohya Y, Ito K. Effects of a short-term parental education program on childhood atopic dermatitis: a randomized controlled trial. Pediatr Dermatol. 2013;30(4):438–43.

38. Ricci G, Bendandi B, Aiazzi R, Patrizi A, Masi M. Educational and medical programme for young children affected by atopic dermatitis and for their parents. Dermatol Psychosom. 2004;5(4):187–92.

39. Brown KK, Rehmus WE, Kimball AB. Determining the relative importance of patient motivations for nonadherence to topical corticosteroid therapy in psoriasis. J Am Acad Dermatol. 2006;55(4):607–13.

40. Chisolm SS, Taylor SL, Balkrishnan R, Feldman SR. Written action plans: potential for improving outcomes in children with atopic dermatitis. J Am Acad Dermatol. 2008;59(4):677–83.

41. Sauder MB, McEvoy A, Sampson M, Kanigsberg N, Vaillancourt R, Ramien ML, et al. The effectiveness of written action plans in atopic dermatitis. Pediatr Dermatol. 2016;33(2):e151–3.

42. Rork JF, Sheehan WJ, Gaffin JM, Timmons KG, Sidbury R, Schneider LC, et al. Parental response to written eczema action plans in children with eczema. Arch Dermatol. 2012;148(3):391–2.

43. Anderson KL, Dothard EH, Huang KE, Feldman SR. Frequency of primary nonadherence to acne treatment. JAMA Dermatol. 2015;151(6):623–6.

44. Yentzer BA, Ade RA, Fountain JM, Clark AR, Taylor SL, Fleischer AB Jr, et al. Simplifying regimens promotes greater adherence and outcomes with topical acne medications: a randomized controlled trial. Cutis. 2010;86(2):103–8.

45. Luersen K, Davis SA, Kaplan SG, Abel TD, Winchester WW, Feldman SR. Sticker charts: a method for improving adherence to treatment of chronic diseases in children. Pediatr Dermatol. 2012;29(4):403–8.

46. Graves MM, Roberts MC, Rapoff M, Boyer A. The efficacy of adherence interventions for chronically ill children: a meta-analytic review. J Pediatr Psychol. 2010;35(4):368–82.

47. Iversen I. Skinner's early research: from reflexology to operative conditioning. Am Psychol. 1992;47:1318–28.

Chapter 6
Adherence in Patients with Comorbidities

Abigail Cline, Adrian Pona, and Steven R. Feldman

Introduction

The association of certain dermatoses and other chronic diseases is complex and multifactorial. Lifestyle factors, impaired health-related quality of life, depression, and therapeutic interventions often confound this relationship. When investigating morbidities in the field of dermatology, psoriasis has received the most attention in the last decades [1]. Epidemiological investigations have largely focused on psoriasis-related conditions such as arthritis, cardiovascular disease, and depression [2]. The search for other comorbidities has now extended to other chronic inflammatory skin diseases, such as rosacea, atopic dermatitis, hidradenitis suppurativa, seborrheic dermatitis, and lichen planus [3–7].

The concepts of multimorbidity and comorbidity have become increasingly important as patients with multiple conditions are becoming the rule rather than the exception. Multimorbidity is the co-existence of two or more chronic conditions [8]. The term comorbidity is now taken to mean a condition with other linked conditions (e.g., diabetes and cardiovascular disease), or when there are conditions that commonly co-exist, (e.g., diabetes and depression). There is greater demand for improving patient outcomes with multiple chronic conditions as health care expenditures are higher in these patients compared to patients with a single chronic disease [8, 9]. One in four American citizens lives with two or more chronic conditions [10]. The prevalence of multimorbidity is estimated to be between 25–55% at 60 years of age and 80% in those older than 75 years [11]. Individuals with multimorbidity are more likely to be admitted to hospital, have longer hospital stays, experience depression, and die prematurely [12, 13]. Nonadherence is highly prevalent in patients with multimorbidity, especially when multiple medications are prescribed for each chronic condition [14].

Despite the increasing number of patients with multiple chronic conditions, evidence on the effectiveness of interventions to increase adherence and improve outcomes in such patients is limited. Whereas different interventions for managing chronic disease have been created, these strategies usually focus only on a single disease [15]. We know very little about the potential impact of interventions for improving adherence in patients managing multiple diseases. This chapter will explore what

A. Cline (✉) · A. Pona
Department of Dermatology, Wake Forest School of Medicine, Winston-Salem, NC, USA
e-mail: aecline@wakehealth.edu

S. R. Feldman
Departments of Dermatology, Pathology and Social Sciences & Health Policy, Wake Forest School of Medicine, Winston-Salem, NC, USA

© Springer Nature Switzerland AG 2020
S. R. Feldman et al. (eds.), *Treatment Adherence in Dermatology*, Updates in Clinical Dermatology, https://doi.org/10.1007/978-3-030-27809-0_6

factors act as barriers to medication adherence in patients with multimorbidities. We also aim to evaluate what interventions may enhance patient adherence to treatment regimens.

Barriers to Adherence in Patients with Multiple Chronic Conditions

Medication Barriers

Patients with multimorbidities face compounded barriers related to their medication, including limited medication access, high medication cost, regimen complexity, noxious side effects, and medication intolerance.

Medication Cost

Patients taking multiple medications tend to incur higher out-of-pocket medication costs, which influences how many medications a patient can afford [16]. Patients also may be reluctant to take multiple medications, with some patients reporting they reached their limit or threshold for taking medication. Adding one more drug to their regimen may not be financially feasible, as one out of five low-income patients do not fill all their prescriptions because of cost. Likewise, patients reported skipping doses to make their prescriptions last longer [17]. Trust also plays a role in medication adherence, as patients with low trust in their physician are more likely to forgo medicines because of cost pressures [18].

Polypharmacy

Medication management for multiple chronic conditions often results in polypharmacy, leading to an increased risk of drug interactions that may result in hospitalization and death [19, 20]. These effects are more pronounced in economically disadvantaged, minority populations with fewer financial resources [21, 22]. Polypharmacy also suggests an underuse of necessary treatments, low adherence, and partly preventable mortality, particularly in older patients [23].

Regimen Complexity

Complex regimens may have conflicting directions, leading to decreased adherence in patients with multiple comorbid conditions [24]. The more medications a patient is required to organize and remember, the poorer the adherence. Infrequent and irregular dosing schedules increase regimen complexity (e.g., large quantities of pills taken only one or twice a week) and decrease the likelihood of adherence. Increases in the number of medications or the number of doses per day results in decreased adherence [25].

Side Effects

Noxious medication side effects or route of medication (e.g., injection) play a strong role in low patient adherence. Adverse medication interactions are more likely to occur as the number of medications increase, contributing to decreased adherence. Patients may actively choose not to take the medications because of negative side effects due to either a specific medication or interactions between medications. Even with topical corticosteroids, as many as 80.7% of patients reported having fears of adverse effects, and 36% admitted to treatment nonadherence due to concern about steroid-related adverse effects [26].

Provider Barriers

Multiple Physicians

Fragmentation of care is a significant problem for patients managing multiple chronic conditions. The involvement of both primary care and multiple specialists can result in too many healthcare providers prescribing medications, too many pharmacies filling prescriptions, and no sharing of information between those entities or with the patient [27]. As the number of prescribing providers and pharmacies increases, patients are less likely to adhere to a medication regimen [24]. Patients with a greater morbidity burden have a higher use of specialists even for conditions that are normally managed in primary care [28]. Interestingly, when a specialist, not a primary care physician, is prescribing the medications, adherence is higher among patients [24].

Physician-Patient Interactions

The physician-patient relationship can influence a patient's decision to adhere to medical recommendations. Issues that may strain the physician-patient relationship and lead to nonadherence include expectations for communication and participation during the clinical encounter, misunderstandings between patients and providers, and different agendas that are not met during clinic visits [29, 30]. When patients report suboptimal communication and relationship with their physicians, they may feel intimidated or disregarded, which often makes it difficult for them to follow the doctor's recommendations. Furthermore, patients report that when their own preferences and goals were not generally integrated into treatment plans, they ended up taking less medication than prescribed [31].

Patient Barriers

Psychiatric Comorbidities

A serious, but often neglected, comorbidity is compromised mental health status. Psoriasis is strongly associated with depression, anxiety, and suicidality [32]. For example, in a recent population-based study, 12.5% of patients with severe psoriasis reported a history of depression, as compared with 4.7% in the control population [33]. Patients with multiple conditions have poorer quality of life, loss of physical functioning, and are more likely to suffer from psychological stress [8, 34, 35]. Mental health disorders, particularly depression, are more prevalent in people with increasing numbers of physical disorders [36]. Patients in whom depression coexists with other medical conditions may be less adherent to medical or behavioral regimens, have more functional impairment, and increased mortality. Patients with psoriasis and depression view the magnitude of treatment benefit as less important compared to patients with only psoriasis. This indifference toward improving their skin condition results in a high risk of nonadherence. In a potentially vicious cycle, nonadherence can result in deteriorated treatment outcome, which might trigger or worsen depression [37]. Although mental disorders often take a back seat to significant multimorbidity, comorbid depression incrementally worsens health compared with depression alone, with any of the chronic diseases alone, and with any combination of chronic diseases without depression [38].

Patient Beliefs

Patients' beliefs of their conditions and medications influence medication adherence, especially in patients with high comorbidity. Some patients may believe that drugs are toxic products which create a vicious cycle, and that spontaneous recovery may occur without treatment. Patients may consider drug prescriptions to be a consequence of a lack of time or resources for other types of treatments. Some patients have identified the pill burden as an excuse by the health system to not individualize treatment. If patients do not perceive therapeutic effectiveness from their treatment, their motivation could decrease and thus hinder adherence. This is particularly significant in patients suffering from several comorbidities who may require lifelong treatment with certain medications [39].

Interventions

Despite the increasing prevalence of patients with multiple chronic conditions, evidence on the effectiveness of interventions to improve clinical outcomes in such patients is limited. Given the complexity of multimorbidity, potential interventions are likely to be complex and multifaceted if they are to address the varied needs of these individuals.

Patient Education

Patient education is the starting point of adherence and nonadherence conduct. Patients' beliefs and misbeliefs influence both intentional and unintentional nonadherence. Patient beliefs of overmedication, lack of satisfactory results following initial expectations, and a fear of side effects can all lead to nonadherence. Cognitive theories such as health belief model and the theory of planned behavior assume that if patients are educated on the benefits and risks of taking medications, they will be better adherent with the medications [40]. Therefore, health professionals can engage with chronic patients, discuss their health beliefs, and provide them with the adequate information about their illness and treatment to increase adherence.

Education is a central element that enables patients to manage their conditions better. In a focus group about multimorbidity and medication adherence, participants stressed the importance of patient education. Participants reported that more information would improve their adherence to the treatment regimens. A lack of knowledge about the therapeutic mechanism and potential adverse effects increased patients' fear of medication and distrust in medicine. Patient confidence in the treatment increased when health providers explained how their medications worked. If patients received adequate information, they showed a clear interest in being involved in decision-making throughout the therapeutic process [39].

Care-Coordination Interventions

Clinical guidelines usually focus on a single disease, so management of multimorbidity can be overwhelming for both patients and providers because of overlapping or conflicting treatments. Care-coordination involves organizing different providers and services to ensure timely and efficient health care delivery. Examples of case-coordination interventions include multidisciplinary teams, case management, and health technology. These interventions focus not only on clinical aspects of care, but also consider patients' health priorities and goals and their social and emotional well-being. In patients with multiple chronic conditions, care-coordination interventions improved cognitive functioning, increased use of mental health services, and reduced symptoms of depression and functional impairment [41].

In dermatology, care-coordination through the use of multidisciplinary clinic practices models have helped provide efficient care have improved outcomes for patients with psoriasis, cutaneous lymphomas, and sarcoidosis [42–44]. The emphasis of care-coordination in dermatology has led to care-coordination as one of the improvement activities considered in the Merit-based Incentive Payment System [45]. While teledermatology has potential to improve care-coordination for patients, fragmentation of care and inadequate follow-up are concerns [46].

Combining educational components with care-coordination interventions appear to have the greatest potential for improving outcomes in patients managing multiple chronic conditions. The combination of case management, education, and self-management significantly reduced depressive symptoms in older adults with multimorbidities. Furthermore, care-coordination or telemedicine interventions with an education component significantly reduced patient disability and improved cognitive functioning [41].

Simplify Regimens

Patients with multimorbidity may have specific problems with medication use that relate to polypharmacy and managing complex treatment regimens. For that reason, interventions targeting specific difficulties related to medication management may be particularly effective. Subjects from the focus group report wanting a therapeutic balance between the dosage schedule and their quality of life. Tailoring treatment regimens to patients' needs and preferences might improve adherence to medication [39]. Reducing the complexity of drug regimens can improve adherence and clinical improvement for some patients, although most of these studies were conducted with single disease conditions [47]. Polymedicated patients want to prioritize drugs regarded as essential for survival and to maintain a good quality of life. From their point of view, doctors should review their medications regularly to see whether they are still necessary [39].

If the number of medications cannot be reduced, then strategies to make treatment regimens and administration are necessary. Packaging interventions such as pill boxes and blister packaging effectively increase medication adherence [48]. Linking medication taking with existing habits also increase medication adherence. Using prompts, such as text messaging, cell phone alarms, and calendars, have also shown promise in helping patients to learn their regimen and remember to take their medications [49].

Patient-Provider Relationship

Patients often report a good relationship with their doctor as the most significant facilitator for adherence [31]. When patients were asked what helped them to follow a treatment or improve medication adherence, responses centered on the attention they received from their prescriber [39]. Patients who feel that their physicians communicate well with them and actively encourage them to be involved in their own care tend to be more motivated to adhere. The amount of contact a patient has with a physician positively correlates with medication adherence [24]. Higher rates of contact with the medical office staff provide more opportunities for medication management and adherence checks.

The greater the patient's confidence in the prescriber, the greater the patient's confidence in the treatment. A strong patient-provider relationship also enhances patient self-care, which in turn improves medication adherence [50]. Many patients report wanting more complete information and education from healthcare providers so as to be more involved in decision-making. When physicians and patients agree on how involved patients should be in their care, adherence is improved [51]. The concept of therapeutic alliance has been largely studied in the field of psychotherapy, where it plays a major role as a good predictor of clinical outcome [52]. It helps both healthcare professionals and patients to work together effectively. The literature has also described the relationship between good medication adherence and therapeutic alliance [53].

Patient participation promotes effective management plans, fosters more effective treatment relationships between patients and providers, and provides the context to explore therapeutic options, discuss medication regimens, and consider follow-up actions [54]. However, patients also complain about the little attention given to mental health status in medical visits. Patients may seek greater clinical support concerning emotional aspects, such as a holistic approach that takes their preferences and family context into account [39].

Treatment of Mental Health Status

It is important to assess the mental health status of patients. Addressing and treating patients' depression may be a neglected opportunity to improve care. The prevalence of psychological comorbidities with multiple chronic conditions is high, so referral to a psychologist or psychiatrist is recommended if psychopathology is noted. While it remains uncertain whether depression management results in increased treatment adherence, depression management can decrease the morbidity associated with other chronic conditions. Sustained depression management program over at least 2 years can diminish the combined effect of multimorbidity and depression on mortality [55].

Conclusion

Understanding medication regimen complexity and lack of shared decision making seem to be major barriers to adherence faced by patients with multimorbidity. Providers should consider interventions aimed at improving care-coordination, patient education, simplifying treatment regimens, and strengthening the provider-patient relationship to help improve patients' adherence to complex medication regimens.

Funding sources None

Conflicts of Interest Dr. Feldman is a speaker for Taro. He is a consultant and speaker for Galderma, Abbvie, Celgene, Abbott Labs, Lilly, Janssen, Novartis Pharmaceuticals and Leo Pharma Inc. Dr. Feldman has received grants from Galderma, Janssen, Abbott Labs, Abbvie, Celgene, Taro, Sanofi, Celgene, Novartis Pharmaceuticals, Qurient, Pfizer Inc. and Anacor. He is a consultant for Advance Medical, Caremark, Gerson Lehrman Group, Guidepoint Global, Kikaku, Lilly, Merck & Co Inc., Mylan, Pfizer Inc., Qurient, Sanofi, Sienna, Sun Pharma, Suncare Research, Valeant, and Xenoport. Dr. Feldman is the founder, chief technology officer and holds stock in Causa Research. Dr. Feldman holds stock and is majority owner in Medical Quality Enhancement Corporation. He receives Royalties from UpToDate, Informa and Xlibris.

Dr. Abigail Cline and Dr. Adrian Pona have no conflicts of interest to disclose.

References

1. Takeshita J, Grewal S, Langan SM, et al. Psoriasis and comorbid diseases: epidemiology. J Am Acad Dermatol. 2017;76(3):377–90.
2. Shah K, Mellars L, Changolkar A, Feldman SR. Real-world burden of comorbidities in US patients with psoriasis. J Am Acad Dermatol. 2017;77:287–292.e4.
3. Haber R, El Gemayel M. Comorbidities in rosacea: a systematic review and update. J Am Acad Dermatol. 2018;78(4):786–92.. e788
4. Andersen YMF, Egeberg A, Skov L, Thyssen JP. Comorbidities of atopic dermatitis: beyond rhinitis and asthma. Curr Dermatol Rep. 2017;6(1):35–41.
5. Dauden E, Lazaro P, Aguilar MD, et al. Recommendations for the management of comorbidity in hidradenitis suppurativa. J Eur Acad Dermatol Venereol. 2018;32(1):129–44.
6. Imamoglu B, Hayta SB, Guner R, Akyol M, Ozcelik S. Metabolic syndrome may be an important comorbidity in patients with seborrheic dermatitis. Arch Med Sci Atheroscler Dis. 2016;1(1):e158–61.
7. Dreiher J, Shapiro J, Cohen AD. Lichen planus and dyslipidaemia: a case-control study. Br J Dermatol. 2009;161(3):626–9.
8. Fortin M, Lapointe L, Hudon C, Vanasse A, Ntetu AL, Maltais D. Multimorbidity and quality of life in primary care: a systematic review. Health Qual Life Outcomes. 2004;2:51.
9. Smith SM, O'Dowd T. Chronic diseases: what happens when they come in multiples? Br J Gen Pract. 2007;57(537):268–70.
10. Anderson G, Horvath J. The growing burden of chronic disease in America. Public Health Rep (Washington, DC: 1974). 2004;119(3):263–70.
11. Fortin M, Stewart M, Poitras ME, Almirall J, Maddocks H. A systematic review of prevalence studies on multimorbidity: toward a more uniform methodology. Ann Fam Med. 2012;10(2):142–51.
12. Deeg DJH, Portrait F, Lindeboom M. Health profiles and profile-specific health expectancies of older women and men: the Netherlands. J Women Aging. 2002;14(1–2):27–46.
13. Bahler C, Huber CA, Brungger B, Reich O. Multimorbidity, health care utilization and costs in an elderly community-dwelling population: a claims data based observational study. BMC Health Serv Res. 2015;15:23.
14. Beusterien KM, Davis EA, Flood R, Howard K, Jordan J. HIV patient insight on adhering to medication: a qualitative analysis. AIDS Care. 2008;20(2):244–52.
15. Ward BW, Schiller JS. Prevalence of multiple chronic conditions among US adults: estimates from the National Health Interview Survey, 2010. Prev Chronic Dis. 2013;10:E65.
16. Mojtabai R, Olfson M. Medication costs, adherence, and health outcomes among Medicare beneficiaries. Health Aff (Project Hope). 2003;22(4):220–9.
17. Safran DG, Neuman P, Schoen C, et al. Prescription drug coverage and seniors: how well are states closing the gap? Health Aff (Project Hope). 2002;Suppl Web Exclusives:W253–68.
18. Piette JD, Heisler M, Krein S, Kerr EA. The role of patient-physician trust in moderating medication nonadherence due to cost pressures. Arch Intern Med. 2005;165(15):1749–55.
19. Winterstein AG, Sauer BC, Hepler CD, Poole C. Preventable drug-related hospital admissions. Ann Pharmacother. 2002;36(7–8):1238–48.
20. Wolff JL, Starfield B, Anderson G. Prevalence, expenditures, and complications of multiple chronic conditions in the elderly. Arch Intern Med. 2002;162(20):2269–76.
21. Kaplan RC, Bhalodkar NC, Brown EJ Jr, White J, Brown DL. Race, ethnicity, and sociocultural characteristics predict noncompliance with lipid-lowering medications. Prev Med. 2004;39(6):1249–55.
22. Shenolikar RA, Balkrishnan R, Camacho FT, Whitmire JT, Anderson RT. Race and medication adherence in Medicaid enrollees with type-2 diabetes. J Natl Med Assoc. 2006;98(7):1071–7.
23. Jyrkka J, Enlund H, Korhonen MJ, Sulkava R, Hartikainen S. Polypharmacy status as an indicator of mortality in an elderly population. Drugs Aging. 2009;26(12):1039–48.
24. Vik SA, Maxwell CJ, Hogan DB. Measurement, correlates, and health outcomes of medication adherence among seniors. Ann Pharmacother. 2004;38(2):303–12.
25. Park DC, Jones TR. Medication adherence and aging. In: Handbook of human factors and the older adult. San Diego: Academic; 1997. p. 257–87.
26. Aubert-Wastiaux H, Moret L, Le Rhun A, et al. Topical corticosteroid phobia in atopic dermatitis: a study of its nature, origins and frequency. Br J Dermatol. 2011;165(4):808–14.
27. Wallace E, Salisbury C, Guthrie B, Lewis C, Fahey T, Smith SM. Managing patients with multimorbidity in primary care. BMJ (Clinical Research Ed). 2015;350:h176.
28. Starfield B, Lemke KW, Herbert R, Pavlovich WD, Anderson G. Comorbidity and the use of primary care and specialist care in the elderly. Ann Fam Med. 2005;3(3):215–22.

29. Britten N, Stevenson FA, Barry CA, Barber N, Bradley CP. Misunderstandings in prescribing decisions in general practice: qualitative study. BMJ (Clinical Research Ed). 2000;320(7233):484–8.

30. Barry CA, Bradley CP, Britten N, Stevenson FA, Barber N. Patients' unvoiced agendas in general practice consultations: qualitative study. BMJ (Clinical Research Ed). 2000;320(7244):1246–50.

31. Mishra SI, Gioia D, Childress S, Barnet B, Webster RL. Adherence to medication regimens among low-income patients with multiple comorbid chronic conditions. Health Soc Work. 2011;36(4):249–58.

32. Van Voorhees AS, Fried R. Depression and quality of life in psoriasis. Postgrad Med. 2009;121(4):154–61.

33. Kurd SK, Troxel AB, Crits-Christoph P, Gelfand JM. The risk of depression, anxiety, and suicidality in patients with psoriasis: a population-based cohort study. Arch Dermatol. 2010;146(8):891–5.

34. Brettschneider C, Leicht H, Bickel H, et al. Relative impact of multimorbid chronic conditions on health-related quality of life–results from the MultiCare Cohort Study. PLoS One. 2013;8(6):e66742.

35. Gunn JM, Ayton DR, Densley K, et al. The association between chronic illness, multimorbidity and depressive symptoms in an Australian primary care cohort. Soc Psychiatry Psychiatr Epidemiol. 2012;47(2):175–84.

36. Barnett K, Mercer SW, Norbury M, Watt G, Wyke S, Guthrie B. Epidemiology of multimorbidity and implications for health care, research, and medical education: a cross-sectional study. Lancet. 2012;380(9836):37–43.

37. Schmieder A, Schaarschmidt ML, Umar N, et al. Comorbidities significantly impact patients' preferences for psoriasis treatments. J Am Acad Dermatol. 2012;67(3):363–72.

38. Moussavi S, Chatterji S, Verdes E, Tandon A, Patel V, Ustun B. Depression, chronic diseases, and decrements in health: results from the World Health Surveys. Lancet. 2007;370(9590):851–8.

39. Pagès-Puigdemont N, Mangues MA, Masip M, et al. Patients' perspective of medication adherence in chronic conditions: a qualitative study. Adv Ther. 2016;33(10):1740–54.

40. Jones CJ, Smith H, Llewellyn C. Evaluating the effectiveness of health belief model interventions in improving adherence: a systematic review. Health Psychol Rev. 2014;8(3):253–69.

41. Kastner M, Cardoso R, Lai Y, et al. Effectiveness of interventions for managing multiple high-burden chronic diseases in older adults: a systematic review and meta-analysis. CMAJ. 2018;190(34):E1004–e1012.

42. Tyler KH, Haverkos BM, Hastings J, et al. The role of an integrated multidisciplinary clinic in the management of patients with cutaneous lymphoma. Front Oncol. 2015;5:136.

43. Cobo-Ibanez T, Villaverde V, Seoane-Mato D, et al. Multidisciplinary dermatology-rheumatology management for patients with moderate-to-severe psoriasis and psoriatic arthritis: a systematic review. Rheumatol Int. 2016;36(2):221–9.

44. Mana J, Rubio-Rivas M, Villalba N, et al. Multidisciplinary approach and long-term follow-up in a series of 640 consecutive patients with sarcoidosis: cohort study of a 40-year clinical experience at a tertiary referral center in Barcelona, Spain. Medicine. 2017;96(29):e7595.

45. Barbieri JS, Miller JJ, Nguyen HP, Forman HP, Bolognia JL, VanBeek MJ. Future considerations for clinical dermatology in the setting of 21st century American policy reform: the Medicare access and Children's health insurance program reauthorization act and the merit-based incentive payment system. J Am Acad Dermatol. 2017;76(6):1206–12.

46. Resneck JS Jr, Abrouk M, Steuer M, et al. Choice, transparency, coordination, and quality among direct-to-consumer telemedicine websites and apps treating skin disease. JAMA Dermatol. 2016;152(7):768–75.

47. Schroeder K, Fahey T, Ebrahim S. Interventions for improving adherence to treatment in patients with high blood pressure in ambulatory settings. Cochrane Database Syst Rev. 2004;2:CD004804.

48. Conn VS, Ruppar TM, Chan KC, Dunbar-Jacob J, Pepper GA, De Geest S. Packaging interventions to increase medication adherence: systematic review and meta-analysis. Curr Med Res Opin. 2015;31(1):145–60.

49. Conn VS, Ruppar TM, Enriquez M, Cooper P. Medication adherence interventions that target subjects with adherence problems: systematic review and meta-analysis. Res Social Adm Pharm. 2016;12(2):218–46.

50. Parchman ML, Zeber JE, Palmer RF. Participatory decision making, patient activation, medication adherence, and intermediate clinical outcomes in type 2 diabetes: a STARNet study. Ann Fam Med. 2010;8(5):410–7.

51. Jahng KH, Martin LR, Golin CE, DiMatteo MR. Preferences for medical collaboration: patient-physician congruence and patient outcomes. Patient Educ Couns. 2005;57(3):308–14.

52. Ardito R, Rabellino D. Therapeutic Alliance and outcome of psychotherapy: historical excursus, measurements, and prospects for research. Front Psychol. 2011;2:270.

53. Sylvia LG, Hay A, Ostacher MJ, et al. Association between therapeutic alliance, care satisfaction, and pharmacological adherence in bipolar disorder. J Clin Psychopharmacol. 2013;33(3):343–50.

54. Van Hecke A, Grypdonck M, Defloor T. A review of why patients with leg ulcers do not adhere to treatment. J Clin Nurs. 2009;18(3):337–49.

55. Gallo JJ, Hwang S, Joo JH, et al. Multimorbidity, depression, and mortality in primary care: randomized clinical trial of an evidence-based depression care management program on mortality risk. J Gen Intern Med. 2016;31(4):380–6.

Chapter 7
Adherence in Psoriasis

Wasim Haidari, Eugenie Y. Quan, Abigail Cline, and Steven R. Feldman

Introduction

Psoriasis is a chronic, immune-mediated skin disease that affects up to 3% of the world population and more than eight million Americans [1]. Regardless of psoriasis severity, nearly 60% of psoriasis patients consider to have a major effect on their quality of life (QoL) [2]. Recent studies provided evidence that psoriasis is a systemic disease with multiple cardiovascular and metabolic comorbidities [3]. Patients experience a negative impact on their physical, emotional, and psychosocial well-being. Many psoriasis patients experience embarrassment, self-consciousness, depression, and may suffer from social isolation [2]. Likewise, the economic burden of psoriasis is high. A systematic review estimated that in 2013, direct psoriasis costs ranged from $51.7 billion to $63.2 billion, the indirect costs ranged from $23.9 billion to $35.4 billion, and medical comorbidities were estimated to cost $36.4 billion [4].

Management of psoriasis can be as complex as the disease itself and should be based on the type and severity of psoriasis. Treatment may involve topical corticosteroids, topical steroid-sparing agents such as vitamin D analogues, retinoids, and tacrolimus, phototherapy, and oral therapy with systemic agents such as methotrexate (MTX) and cyclosporine, or treatment with biologic agents. Multifaceted treatment approach may be required to manage complicated disease. However, the complexity of such treatment plans may hinder treatment adherence. Up to 40% of patients self-report that they do not take their medication as directed [5, 6]; moreover, self-report tends to underestimate true nonadherence rates. A 10% decrease in adherence can correspond with a worsening of psoriasis by one point on a nine-point scale [7]. Since nonadherence may explain suboptimal treatment responses, a solution may be to assess and improve adherence prior to escalating therapy.

W. Haidari (✉) · E. Y. Quan
Center for Dermatology Research, Department of Dermatology,
Wake Forest School of Medicine, Winston-Salem, NC, USA
e-mail: whaidari@wakehealth.edu

A. Cline
Department of Dermatology, Wake Forest School of Medicine, Winston-Salem, NC, USA

S. R. Feldman
Departments of Dermatology, Pathology and Social Sciences & Health Policy, Wake Forest School of Medicine, Winston-Salem, NC, USA

© Springer Nature Switzerland AG 2020   59
S. R. Feldman et al. (eds.), *Treatment Adherence in Dermatology*, Updates in Clinical Dermatology,
https://doi.org/10.1007/978-3-030-27809-0_7

Higher rates of adherence correlate with improved clinical response. Bettering treatment adherence has the potential to considerably improve treatment outcome as well as patients' QoL and possibly help control the systemic effects as well. This chapter will assess the prevalence of nonadherence in psoriasis patients, look into nonadherence associated with various treatment modalities, discuss barriers to adherence, and suggest interventions, which may improve psoriasis treatment adherence.

Prevalence of Nonadherence in Psoriasis

It is difficult to determine the prevalence of nonadherence in psoriasis because adherence rates vary widely depending on the methodology used for evaluation (Table 7.1). In a systematic review on non-adherence in psoriasis, adherence rates on average were around 50–60% in clinical trials; however, studies using objective measures of adherence often had much lower rates of adherence compared to studies using subjective measures [8]. Objective measures of adherence include pharmacy fill rates as a measure of primary adherence, and pill counts, medication weights, and electronic monitoring systems as measures of secondary adherence.

Psoriasis patients had the lowest rate of primary adherence compared to other chronic dermatologic conditions, with 44% of psoriasis patients failing to fill their prescriptions [9]. In a study assessing adherence to both topical and oral psoriasis treatments, mean medication adherence was 60.6% when assessed by pill count and medication weight while self-reported adherence rates by patient interview were 92.0%. [10] Both self-reported measures and medication weights tend to overestimate adherence rates compared to electronic monitoring [6]. Electronic monitoring may consists of a microchip installed into the medication cap to record the opening and closing of the bottles. Electronic monitoring measured an adherence rate of 67% compared to 92% as recorded by psoriasis patient diaries [11].

Adherence rates also vary widely depending on treatment modality. In a self-reported questionnaire, adherence rates were 100% for biologics, 96% for oral medications, 93% for phototherapy, and 75% for topical therapies; however, these rates are likely inflated given that the measurements were self-reported and subjective [12].

Nonadherence to Specific Treatments

Nonadherence to Topical Treatments

Topical treatments are associated with the lowest adherence rates. While 77% of surveyed patients reported nonadherence overall, topical treatments had the highest nonadherence rate (97%), with lack of treatment efficacy cited most frequently as the reason for nonadherence [13]. A systematic review on adherence to topical psoriasis treatments showed frequency of applications varying between 50% and 60% of those expected. Patients also applied between 35% and 72% of the prescribed dose [14]. Long-term adherence rates are even lower compared to short-term rates. Adherence to topical psoriasis medications decreased from 84.6% initially to 51% at the end of the 8 weeks [15]. In a study using electronic monitoring of topical treatment over the course of 12 months, patients used no treatment 37.4% of the days in the first month. By the twelfth month, patients used no treatment to 50.9% of the days. Drug holidays of 7 days or more were common, with a rate of 35.2% of subjects in the first month, increasing to 42.8% of subjects in the twelfth month [16].

Table 7.1 Prevalence of nonadherence in psoriasis

Study	Sample size	Psoriasis treatment evaluated	Measure of adherence	Key results
Zaghloul et al. [10]	N = 201	Topical and oral treatment	Pill count and medication weight of topical therapy were used to objectively measure medication adherence.	The overall mean medication adherence was 60.6%
Carroll et al. [15]	N = 30	Topical therapy	Adherence was measured using 3 methods of adherence monitoring: electronic monitoring caps; medication logs; and medication usage by weight.	Adherence rates calculated from the medication logs and medication weights were consistently higher than those of the electronic monitors (P < 0.05). Electronically measured adherence rates declined from 84.6% to 51% during the 8-week study (P < 0.0001).
Storm et al. [9]	N = 86	Topical and oral treatment	Patients were searched using EMR and looked up in the national electronic pharmacy register.	44.2% (N = 38) of psoriasis patients failed to pick up their prescription.
Lynde et al. [48]	N = 75	Narrow-band UVB phototherapy	Adherence was measured by monitoring if patients followed up tor receive their narrow-band UVB phototherapy treatment	Only 21.6% of patients were adherent 80% of the time to phototherapy sessions.
Esposito et al. [38]	N = 650	(TNF)-α blockers, acitretin, and cyclosporine	Data was collected from digital databases and/or medical records.	Retention rate, the proportion of patients who maintain the same drug in a given time period, at month 24 was 81.4 (±3.2) for (TNF)-α blockers compared to methotrexate (61.5% ± 4.3), acitretin (52.2% ± 1.0), and cyclosporine (28.6% ± 2.7).
Doshi et al. [39]	N = 2707	Biologics (adalimumab, etanercept, infliximab, and ustekinumab)	Analysis was performed using Medicare Chronic Condition Data Warehouse files	During the 12 month follow-up, 38% of patients on biologics (adalimumab, etanercept, infliximab, and ustekinumab) were adherent and 46% discontinued treatment.
Alinia et al. [16]	N = 40	Topical fluocinonide	Adherence was measured using electronic monitoring.	In the first month, no medication was used on 37.4% of the days; over the last month of treatment (month 12), no medication was used on 50.9% of the days. Drug holidays of 7 days or more without using treatment were common, occuring in 35.2% of subjects in the first month and 42.8% in the 12th month of study.
Dommasch et al. [34]	N = 22,742	Adalimumab, etanercept, ustekinumab, acitretin, and methotrexate	Adherence was measured by using a proportion of patients, dichotomized as adherent (≥0.80) or nonadherent (<0.80).	Among new users of systemic medications, adherence to adalimumab, etanercept, and ustekinumab was greater and acitretin lower compared with methotrexate.

EMR Electronic Medical Records, *UVB* Ultravioler B, *TNF-α* Tumor necrosis factor-alpha

Low adherence rates are similar between different topical treatments—50% with topical steroids, 57% with vitamin D derivatives, 41% with salicylic acid agents [14]. Commonly cited reasons for poor adherence to topical treatments include low efficacy, increased time consumption with application, and poor cosmetic characteristics of the specific preparation. Similarly, a patient survey conducted on 1291 psoriasis patients throughout Europe found that reasons for nonadherence included poor cosmetic characteristics (29%), low efficacy (27%), increased time consumption (26%), and occurrence of side effects (15%) [17]. Slow absorption (44%), increased application frequency required (41%), staining of clothes (34%) and bedding (27%) were reasons frequently cited in a review of topical medication adherence [18]. In another patient survey conducted on 103 Turkish patients, respondents felt they were too busy (25%), fed up (22%), inadequately educated about the disease and its treatment (20%), forgetful (9%), or treatments were too costly (5%) [19]. In a small survey of 50 Korean patients, 18% of patients felt that their topical treatment was moderately or very unpleasant because of its cosmetic characteristics (e.g. odor, texture), 40% considered their treatment to be costly, and 40% were concerned about the adverse effects of treatment. 81.8% of patients cited forgetfulness as the primary reason for nonadherence, 18.8% cited unclear instructions, and 10% reported inconvenience and concerns about side effects [20]. Adherence improved with higher efficacy treatments, treatments that were less greasy, sticky, or smelly, and treatments with a lower risk of side effects [14].

Topical Corticosteroids

Even though topical corticosteroids are the mainstay of topical psoriasis treatment, patients may hesitate to use them. In a patient questionnaire on adherence to topical corticosteroids in psoriasis patients, 60% of respondents were fearful of side effects and 42% reported avoiding prescription medications unless they felt it was absolutely necessary. Similar to the reasons for nonadherence to topical treatments overall, efficacy, time, formulation, and cost all contributed to low adherence to topical corticosteroids, with 15% of patients surveyed attributing their nonadherence to the product being "too messy/oily/sticky" and 10% citing increased frequency of application required through the day [21]. Dissatisfaction with efficacy, inconvenient or unpleasant treatment, undesirable cosmetic properties (e.g. greasy, desiccating, sticky, or smelly vehicles), and fear of adverse drug effects were common reasons for nonadherence to topical corticosteroids repeatedly cited in multiple studies [12, 14, 17, 22, 23]. Although ointment formulations are more efficacious when applied as prescribed, overall low adherence given the poor cosmetic characteristics and inconvenience with application results in suboptimal treatment outcomes [24]. Different formulations, such as foams and sprays, are more likely to have greater patient acceptance, consequently translating to greater adherence and improved treatment outcomes. Prices of topical corticosteroids, including generic preparations, are dramatically rising—a single tube of product can cost several hundred dollars. Significantly increasing cost of treatment is also likely to contribute to nonadherence [25].

Vitamin D Analogues

Topical vitamin D analogues for treatment of psoriasis are as effective as mid-potency corticosteroids and include calcipotriol, calcitriol, and tacalcitol. Skin irritation is a commonly reported side effect. In a randomized, single-blinded study involving 75 psoriasis patients comparing the safety and efficacy of calcitriol and calcipotriol, calcitriol was associated with decreased rates of perilesional erythema and edema, stinging, and burning. Irritant and contact dermatitis were adverse effects only seen in patients treated with calcipotriol [26]. Combined use of topical vitamin D analogues and corticosteroids is more effective than either agent alone; the anti-inflammatory effects of the topical corticosteroid reduce the irritation caused by the vitamin D analogue, while the vitamin D analogue acts as a corticosteroid-sparing agent and reduces corticosteroid-specific side effects [27]. Calcipotriol-betamethasone dipropionate compound therapy was more effective and better tolerated than either placebo, calcipotriol, or betamethasone alone. Patients in the study reported ease of use (95.2%), good skin absorption (77.7%), good cosmetic characteristics of the vehicle (74.3%), decreased time consumption (73.4%), and little interference with social activities (68.4%) as reasons for adherence [28].

Calcineurin Inhibitors

Calcineurin inhibitors are effective for treatment of psoriasis in sensitive areas and include topical tacrolimus and pimecrolimus. Both medications are generally well-tolerated; the most common side effects reported include burning, stinging, hyperesthesia, and itching [29]. There is a FDA-issued black box warning based on a theoretical risk of lymphoma and skin cancer with topical calcineurin inhibitor use. No definite causal relationship has been established and further studies have not found any evidence of an associated increased risk of malignancy; however, this may decrease adherence rates as fear of adverse effects is a commonly cited reason for nonadherence [30].

Tazarotene

Tazarotene, a topical retinoid, is an effective treatment option for psoriasis; however, its use is limited by its adverse effects, including pruritus, burning, stinging, erythema, irritation, dermatitis, and desquamation [31]. Concomitant treatment with a topical corticosteroid reduces irritation and can improve adherence rates [32].

Tar

While not a first-line therapy for psoriasis, tar-based treatments can be a helpful adjunct to topical corticosteroids. Many patients, however, do not find tar-based treatments to be cosmetically acceptable and often find products to be messy with an unpleasant odor. Topical tar preparations can also stain hair, skin, and clothing [33].

Nonadherence to Systemic Therapies

Moderate-to-severe psoriasis frequently requires long-term systemic therapy. As with topical treatments, multiple factors such as efficacy, safety, and patient's overall satisfaction with treatment affect adherence. A recent retrospective, comparative cohort study studied adherence of new users of acitretin, adalimumab, etanercept, MTX, and ustekinumab using a large US health insurance claims database. Among the 22,472 new users of systemic medications, adherence to adalimumab, etanercept, and ustekinumab was greater and acitretin lower compared to MTX [34]. These results were consistent with prior studies using data outside US, which have shown greater adherence to biologics compared to other systemic agents [34].

Drug survival may also serve as an indicator of therapeutic success. A study assessing drug survival rates and reasons for discontinuation demonstrated that the crude probability for drug survival in patients with moderate-to-severe psoriasis was higher for biologics (ustekinumab, followed by adalimumab, etanercept, infliximab) than of traditional systemic therapies (MTX, acitretin, and cyclosporine A). Inefficacy with respect to cutaneous lesions was the reason for discontinuing biologics with the exception of infliximab, which along with traditional systemic antipsoriatic agents, were most frequently discontinued to adverse events [35]. A study looking at retention rate, the proportion of patients who maintain the same drug in a given time period, revealed that global retention rate of (TNF)-α blockers at month 24 was 81.4% (±3.2) compared to MTX (61.5% ± 4.3), acitretin (52.2% ± 1.0), and cyclosporine (28.6% ± 2.7) [38]. Long-term treatment of psoriasis patients should integrate the current knowledge of drug survival rates when making therapeutic decisions.

Biologics

Psoriasis patient adherence to biological treatments is challenging. Psoriasis patients appear to have the highest adherence with biological therapy. In Medicaid-enrolled patients, adherence rates were highest for biologics (66%) compared to other psoriasis treatments which included topical, oral/systemic agents, and phototherapy (36%) [36]. The overall pharmacy claim rates for biologics were 61.9% compared to 50.7% for MTX [34]. Injectable drugs are often preferred over orally administered medicine [37]. This may contribute to increased adherence of injectable biologics compared to oral medications. Positive feedback on adherence due to the high efficacy of biologics in psoriasis patients may contribute to the long-term adherence to these drugs. Patients on biologics also usually suffer from a more severe form of psoriasis compared to patients using topical therapy or phototherapy. In theory, this might result in higher motivation and hence treatment adherence among those on biologics, but patients with more severe psoriasis may have worse adherence than those with milder disease [10, 12]. Drug survival time was also longer for biologics than for oral agents [35]. In a retrospective study, biologics targeting tumor necrosis factor (TNF)-α had a 72.6% adherence rate after 30 months of treatment [38].

However, psoriasis patients continue to have poor adherence to biologics. In a retrospective claims analysis of 2009 through 2012 data from Medicare patients, 2707 patients initiating adalimumab (40%), etanercept (37.9%), infliximab (11.7%), and ustekinumab (10.3%) were examined. During the 12-month follow-up, 38% of patients were adherent and 46% discontinued treatment [39]. In another study, ustekinumab had a higher adherence rate compared to other biologic agents. In biologic-naïve and biologic experienced psoriasis patients, the drug survival of ustekinumab was better than adalimumab and etanercept [34]. Better adherence to ustekinumab was also supported by an Australian study on the use of biological therapies in psoriasis in real-life clinical setting; approximately 90% of patients remained on ustekinumab treatment after almost 3 years [40]. Reasons for nonadherence to biologics may include fear of side effects and high cost of treatment.

Methotrexate

In psoriasis, MTX is an anti-inflammatory medication; it increases endogenous anti-inflammatory adenosine levels. MTX is effective for psoriasis. Approximately 40% of patients on MTX achieve 75% improvement in Psoriasis Area and Severity Index (PASI 75) if provided as continuous therapy over 4-month period at reasonable dosing [41]. Although an effective medication for psoriasis, the efficacy of MTX is lower compared to most biologic agents. Severe adverse events such as pancytopenia, hepatotoxicity, and pulmonary fibrosis and less serious side effects such as nausea and vomiting may occur with MTX therapy [41]. Fear of potential side effects may contribute to nonadherence to MTX.

Few studies have examined the overall adherence of MTX in psoriasis patients. A study looking at retention rate revealed that retention rate for MTX was lower than that of TNF-α blockers at 24 and

30 months (p < 0.001) [42]. There is also a difference between adherence to oral and subcutaneous (SC) MTX. To further investigate this, one study assessed the adherence of SC MTX in a multicenter retrospective analysis of chronic plaque-type psoriasis patient registry. Adherence to self-administered SC MTX after 6 months of treatment was high. Most patients who were switched to SC MTX after an unsuccessful treatment with oral MTX remained on subcutaneous regimen [43].

Cyclosporine

Dermatologists may use cyclosporine to treat extensive or disabling psoriasis when rapid response is desired. In psoriasis, cyclosporine works by blocking interleukin (IL)-2 and other proinflammatory cytokines and by preventing T-cell activation. Better treatment response is seen in patients receiving highest dosage, and higher doses are also related to increased risk of renal toxicity, hypertension, and intolerability [41].

Although cyclosporine is more useful as a rescue drug than long-term psoriasis treatment, fear of side effects may cause suboptimal adherence even with short-term use. Retention rate of cyclosporine at months 24 and 30 was also lower than retention rate of TNF-α blockers (p < 0.001) and discontinuation was mainly due to intolerance, which was also true for conventional drugs MTX and acitretin [42].

Acitretin

Acitretin is the most widely used retinoid in psoriasis treatment and effective both as monotherapy and combination therapy with conventional systemic drugs as well as biologics. As monotherapy, it's highly efficacious in specific clinical subtypes of psoriasis such as erythrodermic psoriasis, palmoplantar psoriasis, and nail psoriasis [44]. In a study evaluating factors associated with drug survival of MTX and acitretin in patients with psoriasis, younger age (p < 0.001) and psoriatic arthritis (p < 0.001) were factors associated with treatment dropout [45]. Acitretin lacks immunosuppressive side effects; the side effects are usually mild and can be minimized with dose titration [44]. These features of acitretin may help patients better adhere to the treatment.

Nonadherence to Light Therapy

Phototherapy is frequently used to treat plaque psoriasis as it is effective, safe, and accessible treatment without any systemic side effects [46]. It counteracts inflammation-induced characteristic pathological changes of psoriasis because ultraviolet radiation induces apoptosis in T-lymphocytes and in keratinocytes in the epidermis. Ultraviolet-B (UVB) treatment is also highly cost-effective [47] which may aid in adherence to treatment. However, use of UVB phototherapy in the office setting can be challenging for patients. Office-administered UVB requires psoriasis patients to visit two to three times per week for 15–25 treatments, which can be a burden for patients. Hurdles include patients taking time off of work, arranging transportation, and paying co-pays. Therefore, it is no wonder that only 21.6% of patients were adherent 80% of the time to phototherapy sessions [48].

A study of moderate-to-severe psoriasis patients assessed adherence to oral acitretin and home UVB therapy over a 12-week period. Patients had better adherence to home UVB therapy than oral acitretin. Easier access and high perception of effectiveness of home phototherapy (96% of patients reporting positive results) may have contributed to the improved adherence of this treatment [49, 75]. Patients treated at home have a lower burden of treatment and evaluate their therapy more positively than patients treated in the outpatient department (P values ≤0.001) [76]. Lower burden could contribute to better adherence to home treatment [77]. In a retrospective observational study conducted to evaluate patient's adherence to a prescribed three-times-per-week treatment protocol of home UVB phototherapy for localized psoriasis, adherence was calculated for each patient by dividing the number of treatments the patient administered by the number of treatment opportunities they had. Among the 18 psoriasis patients, median continuous adherence was 81% [78].

Barriers to Adherence

In a series of patient interviews, there were several major themes that emerged surrounding the issue of nonadherence in psoriasis. Patients often perceived psoriasis and its treatment as a burden and social stigma, limiting their ability to engage in social activities and balance their work commitments. Poor control of symptoms and unpredictable response to treatment in addition to the perception of psoriasis as a lifelong chronic condition worsened adherence by causing psychological stress and feelings of frustration and hopelessness. Patients often did not feel empathy from healthcare providers and felt that providers rarely acknowledged the challenges associated with medication use. There is some degree of bias in these responses, however, as patients were recruited from psoriasis support groups [50]. Primary drivers of poor adherence in the treatment of skin conditions overall include a poor doctor-patient relationship, lack of knowledge about the disease and treatment, lack of belief in the treatment, unrealistic expectations, side effects or fear of side effects, messy and complex treatment regimens, inadequate follow-up, forgetfulness, psychosocial factors, and cost [51]. Barriers impacting adherence to psoriasis range from education, perception of treatment effectiveness, poor communication, forgetfulness, and poor accountability as well as high cost of treatment.

Fears of Adverse Effects

In a study assessing adherence to conventional systemic and biologic therapies in a real-world setting among psoriasis patients, factors associated with intentional nonadherence included being on conventional systemic therapy, *having strong medication concerns*, weaker routine for taking their systemic therapy, and long treatment duration. Overall 22.4% of patients out of the total sample ($N = 811$) using self-administered systemic therapies were classified as non-adherent [50]. Another study surveying physicians and psoriasis patients determined that inconvenience and *concern about side effects* were common reasons for topical treatment discontinuation. More than 40% of total patients ($N = 50$) surveyed were moderately or very concerned about side effects of topical treatment [20]. Adequately assuring patients about the safety of the drug and explaining that the large majority of patients do not experience the rare side effects may be one approach to address this.

Poor Communication and Knowledge Gaps

The survey study of psoriasis patients using topical treatments also determined that more than 15% of patients did not get enough information about the drug although the majority were satisfied with the length of consultations [20]. This may indicate the possibility that the information was shared with the patients, but it was not sufficient or the patients did not necessarily understand the information conveyed to them and had unanswered questions. Helping patients have a better understanding of their medicine may improve treatment adherence. Another study exploring perceptions of psoriasis patients on their disease and its management revealed that medication underuse was caused by concerns about potential side effects, perceived poor control of symptoms, and feelings of anxiety [50]. Inadequate knowledge about the disease and therapy was listed as a reason for missing treatment by 20% of 103 psoriasis patients in a different study [27]. These findings highlight the importance of patient education and good communication between patients and their physicians.

Forgetfulness

Forgetfulness is a common cause of unintentional nonadherence among psoriasis patients as in many other diseases requiring long-term treatment [27, 52]. Useful strategies to address this problem may include reminders such as text messages or phone calls [53]. Having nurses and other healthcare staff more involved with psoriasis patients may help improve treatment adherence by helping with treatment reminders and also being available to instruct patients on how to apply medications and providing important information about disease when patients have develop questions [54].

High Medication Cost

Increasing costs of psoriasis treatment may also contribute to suboptimal adherence. Biologics are an essential part of treatment regimen for many patients suffering from psoriasis. However, this treatment modality may be very costly [55]. In a large, multinational, population-based survey of psoriasis and psoriatic arthritis patients in Europe and North America involving 3426 subjects, 11% of patients attributed cost/insurance reimbursement issues as the reason for their discontinuation and secondary nonadherence [56]. Low income has a negative impact on adherence as patients may not be able to afford expensive medications [57]. Making medications more affordable and patient assistance programs that provide financial support may be solutions to help combat this adherence barrier.

Adherence Interventions for Psoriasis

There are three key issues that need to be addressed when trying to improve adherence—improving the doctor-patient relationship, increasing the patient's optimism regarding the prescribed treatment, and limiting the "nuisance value" of the treatment in terms of hassle and side effects [5]. Interventions that were the most successful actively engaged the patient and held them accountable for adherence to treatment [51]. Practical strategies to improve adherence then include strengthening the physician-patient relationship, choosing treatments patients are willing to use, providing detailed education about the disease and treatment, and scheduling regular follow-ups [58] (Table 7.2).

Patient Education

Lack of education and information about treatment is associated with low adherence rates [53, 54]. In an analysis of 767 topical psoriasis prescriptions written by both dermatologists and general practitioners, 64.3% of prescriptions were not adequately written and did not have the required information to allow patients to manage their psoriasis treatment correctly [59]. In a patient survey regarding

Table 7.2 Studies reporting adherence intervention in psoriasis patients

Study	Sample size	Intervention to increase adherence	Therapy	Length	Measure of adherence	Adherence result
Balato et al. [69]	N = 20	Intervention group received daily text messages, with medication reminders sent out 3 times weekly and educational tools sent out 4 times weekly.	Biologics, Methotrexate, Acitretin, Cyclosporine	12 weeks	Self-reported	Rates of adherence improved from 3.86 days/week to 6.46 days/week after intervention compared to no change in the control group.
Alinia et al. [16]	N = 40	Internet-based reporting intervention vs. standard-of-care. Intervention group reported their impression of the state of their psoriasis over the internet on a weekly basis.	Topical fluocinonide	12 months	Electronic monitoring	Although not statistically significant, intervention group increased adherence. Overall, 35% of the prescribed number of doses were taken by the control group and 50% for the intervention group (P = 0 08).
Alpalhão et al. [68]	N = 236	Interventional group received three MPCs over a 6-months period (weeks 2, 8, and 16 of the study protocol) and a control group that received none.	Topical and systemic treatment	6 months	Self-reported adherence questionnaires	Although there were no differences in adherence between the treatment and control groups, the proportion of patients who applied the topical medications exactly as prescribed was higher in the phone call group (82.4%) compared to the control (67.4%).
Svendsen et al. [70]	N = 122	Patients were randomized to no app or app intervention groups. Intervention group received daily reminder messages associated with an alert sound as well as additional educational materials available through the application.	Calcipotriol/ betamethasone dipropionate (Cal/BD) foam	22 weeks	Electronic monitoring	65% of participants using the application had high rates of adherence, as measured by medications applied for greater than 80% of the days in a treatment period, compared to 38% of participants in the control group in a 4-week treatment period

MPC Motivational Phone Call

questions on topical treatments, 30% of the questions submitted were related to the safety of topical medications, 16% were on proper use of topical medications, and 11% were on treatment efficacy, demonstrating the need for detailed information and written instructions on prescribed treatments, reference materials for use at home, and educational programs [60]. In a systematic review of adherence to topical psoriasis treatments, patients most frequently desired more information on psoriasis flare triggers, co-morbidities associated with psoriasis, treatment options and their side effects, approximate timeframe of therapy, expected results from therapy, and written instructions on medication use [14]. Not only can the physician take care to express empathy and recognition of the social impact of psoriasis, the physician can also come to a mutual agreement about the treatment plan with the patient and consider implementing an individualized education program, taking into account patient preferences [14].

Patient education can involve both verbal education and written information, group-based learning, audio and videotapes, computer-assisted education, and internet forums and programs [61, 62]. In a randomized controlled study, patients participated in a "Topical Treatment Optimization Program" (TTOP) which consisted of five elements—structured guidance via visit checklist for conversations between the dermatologist and patient and between the nurse and patient, patient information materials, telephone and email help desk, and treatment reminders by phone calls with a nurse. From week 8–64 of treatment with topical calcipotriol-betamethasone, patients in the intervention group consistently demonstrated increased improvements in severity compared to the control, although there were no differences in quality of life measures. Patients in the intervention group also reported feeling more confident and informed about the disease with higher rates of treatment satisfaction by patient survey. Of the five elements, patients ranked the one-on-one conversations with the dermatologist and nurse as the most helpful and important and the help desk and reminder calls as the least important [63].

In another study, patients treated with calcipotriol/betamethasone gel were given extensive information on psoriasis and instructions on application of the medication for 20 minutes. Patients in the intervention group received an additional 20 minutes of individualized training, where the patient applied the medication in the presence of trained staff and received feedback on how much medication to use and how to correctly apply the medication. Patients in the intervention group demonstrated increased improvement in disease severity and increased adherence rates as determined by medication weight [64]. Similarly, interdisciplinary training with information about the treatment and demonstrations on the correct use and application of medications improved adherence by self-reported questionnaire [65]. Psoriasis patients in China demonstrated greater improvement in self-reported adherence after participating in a verbal education program on psoriasis, the appropriate use of medication, and the consequences of poor adherence [66].

Reminders

Implementing a reminder system using telephone calls or text messages to increase accountability can improve adherence. In a meta-analysis of 11 randomized controlled trials, 8 of the 11 studies showed an increase in adherence in the reminder group treatment arm compared to the control [67]. In a randomized controlled trial, patients received 3 motivational phone calls over a 6-month period. Although there were no differences in adherence between the treatment and control groups, the proportion of patients who applied the topical medications exactly as prescribed was higher in the phone call group (82.4%) compared to the control (67.4%) [68]. In a pilot study, patients who received daily text messages, with medication reminders sent out 3 times weekly and educational tools sent out 4 times weekly over a 12-week period, had improved rates of adherence from 3.86 days/week to 6.46 days/week after intervention compared to no change in the control group. Patients who received the text messages also had greater improvements in psoriasis severity and QoL and reported a stronger physician-patient relationship [69].

With the widespread use of smartphones, smartphone applications can be created to improve accountability. An application able to synchronize with an electronic monitoring unit was able to provide feedback on appropriate use of the prescribed psoriasis medication. Patients also received daily reminder messages associated with an alert sound and were able to record their daily treatment in a patient diary within the application. Additional educational materials were also available through the application. 65% of participants using the application had high rates of adherence, as measured by medications applied for greater than 80% of the days in a treatment period, compared to 38% of participants in the control group in a 4-week treatment period [70].

Timing of Follow-Up

Adherence improves in the days immediately before and after office visits [7]. Because adherence declines rapidly after an office visit, scheduling a follow-up visit shortly after starting therapy may improve initial adherence. With greater initial efficacy due to increased initial adherence, patients may feel encouraged to continue with their treatments as prescribed to maintain good control of their disease.

Electronic follow-up is more convenient and potentially could replace in-person office visits. In an investigator-blinded, randomized, prospective study, psoriasis patients on topical therapy used an internet-based reporting system to submit weekly impressions of their psoriasis progress. Although not statistically significant, greater adherence as measured by electronic monitoring was seen in the intervention group (50%) as compared to the control group (30%), with the largest effects on adherence seen within the first month of treatment. The intervention group also had greater improvements in psoriasis severity compared to the control [16].

Multidisciplinary Approach

Efforts to improve adherence should involve a multidisciplinary approach with patient collaboration. In a systematic review of adherence in psoriasis, overall patient satisfaction or satisfaction with the physician-patient relationship, treatment, and quality of care, was associated with higher adherence. Two studies in the review reported the emergence of patient satisfaction as a significant predictor of adherence [6]. It is important to take patient preferences into consideration when coming up with a treatment plan. A study on the concordance between patient preferences and recommended treatments found that patients were willing to accept adverse effects of treatment in exchange for treatment attributes (e.g. treatment duration, frequency, cost) that more closely matched with their personal and professional life [71]. Using the simplest possible therapy, such as prescribing a sustained-release formulation and minimizing frequency of doses required through the day, improves adherence and patient satisfaction [72]. Multiple studies have shown increased adherence with a once daily treatment regimen compared to a twice daily regimen [10, 14].

Including a psychiatrist or psychologist on the multidisciplinary team may be helpful. Several studies have noted the negative impact of psychological issues (e.g. depression, anxiety, resignation, denial) on adherence, while positive attitudes toward treatment and acceptance of the disease increase adherence [73, 74].

Conclusion

While there is no absolute cure for psoriasis, novel therapies allow for substantial reduction in symptoms and considerable improvement in QoL. These treatments will only work if patients adhere to them as recommended by their physicians. Nonadherence is prevalent among psoriasis patients due to fear of adverse effects, knowledge gaps, forgetfulness, and high medication cost. It is important for healthcare providers to appreciate the prevalence of nonadherence in psoriasis and the impact this has on treatment outcomes. Helpful interventions include patient education, improving accountability, early follow-up, and multidisciplinary approach. Improving adherence will certainly lead to better treatment outcomes, reduced suffering, and better quality of life.

Disclosures Feldman has received research, speaking and/or consulting support from a variety of companies including Galderma, GSK/Stiefel, Almirall, Leo Pharma, Boehringer Ingelheim, Mylan, Celgene, Pfizer, Valeant, Abbvie, Samsung, Janssen, Lilly, Menlo, Merck, Novartis, Regeneron, Sanofi, Novan, Qurient, National Biological Corporation, Caremark, Advance Medical, Sun Pharma, Suncare Research, Informa, UpToDate and National Psoriasis Foundation. He is founder and majority owner of www.DrScore.com and founder and part owner of Causa Research, a company dedicated to enhancing patients' adherence to treatment..

Wasim Haidari, Eugenie Quan, and Dr. Cline have no conflicts to disclose.

References

1. Ventura A, Mazzeo M, Gaziano R, Galluzzo M, Bianchi L, Campione E. New insight into the pathogenesis of nail psoriasis and overview of treatment strategies. Drug Des Devel Ther. 2017;11:2527–35.
2. Armstrong AW, Schupp C, Wu J, Bebo B. Quality of life and work productivity impairment among psoriasis patients: findings from the National Psoriasis Foundation survey data 2003–2011. PLoS One. 2012;7(12):e52935.
3. Ryan C, Kirby B. Psoriasis is a systemic disease with multiple cardiovascular and metabolic comorbidities. Dermatol Clin. 2015;33:41–55.
4. Brezinski EA, Dhillon JS, Armstrong AW. Economic burden of psoriasis in the United States: a systematic review. JAMA Dermatol. 2015;151(6):651–8.
5. Richards HL, Fortune DG, Griffiths CE. Adherence to treatment in patients with psoriasis. J Eur Acad Dermatol Venereol. 2006;20(4):370–9.
6. Thorneloe RJ, Bundy C, Griffiths CE, Ashcroft DM, Cordingley L. Adherence to medication in patients with psoriasis: a systematic literature review. Br J Dermatol. 2013;168(1):20–31.
7. Carroll CL, Feldman SR, Camacho FT, Balkrishnan R. Better medication adherence results in greater improvement in severity of psoriasis. Br J Dermatol. 2004;151(4):895–7.
8. Augustin M, Holland B, Dartsch D, Langenbruch A, Radtke MA. Adherence in the treatment of psoriasis: a systematic review. Dermatology. 2011;222(4):363–74.
9. Storm A, Andersen SE, Benfeldt E, Serup J. One in 3 prescriptions are never redeemed: primary non-adherence in an outpatient clinic. J Am Acad Dermatol. 2008;59(1):27–33.
10. Zaghloul SS, Goodfield MJ. Objective assessment of compliance with psoriasis treatment. Arch Dermatol. 2004;140(4):408–14.
11. Balkrishnan R, Carroll CL, Camacho FT, Feldman SR. Electronic monitoring of medication adherence in skin disease: results of a pilot study. J Am Acad Dermatol. 2003;49(4):651–4.
12. Chan SA, Hussain F, Lawson LG, Ormerod AD. Factors affecting adherence to treatment of psoriasis: comparing biologic therapy to other modalities. J Dermatolog Treat. 2013;24(1):64–9.
13. Kivelevitch DN, Tahhan PV, Bourren P, et al. Self-medication and adherence to treatment in psoriasis. Int J Dermatol. 2012;51(4):416–9.
14. Devaux S, Castela A, Archier E, et al. Adherence to topical treatment in psoriasis: a systematic literature review. J Eur Acad Dermatol Venereol. 2012;26(Suppl 3):61–7.
15. Carroll CL, Feldman SR, Camacho FT, et al. Adherence to topical therapy decreases during the course of an 8-week psoriasis clinical trial: commonly used methods of measuring adherence to topical therapy overestimate actual use. J Am Acad Dermatol. 2004;51(2):212–6.

16. Alinia H, Moradi Tuchayi S, Smith JA, et al. Long-term adherence to topical psoriasis treatment can be abysmal: a 1-year randomized intervention study using objective electronic adherence monitoring. Br J Dermatol. 2017;176(3):759–64.

17. Fouere S, Adjadj L, Pawin H. How patients experience psoriasis: results from a European survey. J Eur Acad Dermatol Venereol. 2005;19(Suppl 3):2–6.

18. Lee IA, Maibach HI. Pharmionics in dermatology: a review of topical medication adherence. Am J Clin Dermatol. 2006;7:231–6.

19. Gokdemir G, Ari S, Koslu A. Adherence to treatment in patients with psoriasis vulgaris: Turkish experience. J Eur Acad Dermatol Venereol. 2008;22:330–5.

20. Choi JW, Kim BR, Youn SW. Adherence to topical therapies for the treatment of psoriasis: surveys of physicians and patients. Ann Dermatol. 2017;29(5):559–64.

21. Feldman SR. Disease burden and treatment adherence in psoriasis patients. Cutis. 2013;92(5):258–63.

22. Brown KK, Rehmus WE, Kimball AB. Determining the relative importance of patient motivations for non-adherence to topical corticosteroid therapy in psoriasis. J Am Acad Dermatol. 2006;55(4):607–13.

23. Feldman SR, Horn EJ, Balkrishnan R, et al. Psoriasis: improving adherence to topical. J Am Acad Dermatol. 2008;59(6):1009–16.

24. Bewley A, Page B. Maximizing patient adherence for optimal outcomes in psoriasis. J Eur Acad Dermatol Venereol. 2011;25(Suppl 4):9–14.

25. Reisfeld PL. How high is up? Generic prices rise. Cutis. 2014;93(1):6–8.

26. Ortonne JP, Humbert P, Nicolas JF, et al. Intra-individual comparison of the cutaneous safety and efficacy of calcitriol 3 microg g(−1) ointment and calcipotriol 50 microg g(−1) ointment on chronic plaque psoriasis localized in facial, hairline, retroauricular or flexural areas. Br J Dermatol. 2003;148(2):326–33.

27. Zschocke I, Mrowietz U, Karakasili E, Reich K. Non-adherence and measures to improve adherence in the topical treatment of psoriasis. J Eur Acad Dermatol Venereol. 2014;28 Suppl 2:4–9.

28. Kontochristopoulos G, Kouris A, Chantzaras A, et al. Improvement of health-related quality of life and adherence to treatment with calcipotriol-betamethasone dipropionate gel in patients with psoriasis vulgaris. An Bras Dermatol. 2016;91(2):160–6.

29. Lebwohl M, Freeman AK, Chapman MS, et al. Tacrolimus ointment is effective for facial and intertriginous psoriasis. J Am Acad Dermatol. 2004;51(5):723–30.

30. Siegfried EC, Jaworski JC, Hebert AA. Topical calcineurin inhibitors and lymphoma risk: evidence update with implications for daily practice. Am J Clin Dermatol. 2013;14(3):163–78.

31. Weinstein GD, Koo JY, Krueger GG, et al. Tazarotene cream in the treatment of psoriasis: Two multicenter, double-blind, randomized, vehicle-controlled studies of the safety and efficacy of tazarotene creams 0.05% and 0.1% applied once daily for 12 weeks. J Am Acad Dermatol. 2003;48(5):760–7.

32. Gollnick H, Menter A. Combination therapy with tazarotene plus a topical corticosteroid for the treatment of plaque psoriasis. Br J Dermatol. 1999;140(Suppl 54):18–23.

33. Blakely K, Gooderham M. Management of scalp psoriasis: current perspectives. Psoriasis (Auckl). 2016;6:33–40.

34. Dommasch ED, Lee MP, Joyce CJ, Garry EM, Gagne JJ. Drug utilization patterns and adherence in patients on systemic medications for the treatment of psoriasis: a retrospective, comparative cohort study. J Am Acad Dermatol. 2018;79(6):1061–1068.e1.

35. Arnold T, Schaarschmidt ML, Herr R, et al. Drug survival rates and reasons for drug discontinuation in psoriasis. J Dtsch Dermatol Ges. 2016;14(11):1089–99.

36. Bhosle MK, Feldman SR, et al. Medication adherence and health care costs associated with biologics in Medicaid-enrolled patients with psoriasis. J Dermatolog Treat. 2006;17(5):294–301.

37. Hsu DY, Gniadecki R. Patient adherence to biologic agents in psoriasis. Dermatology. 2016;232(3):326–33.

38. Esposito M, Gisondi P, Cassano N, et al. Survival rate of antitumour necrosis factor-alpha treatments for psoriasis in routine dermatological practice: a multicentre observational study. Br J Dermatol. 2013;169(3):666–72.

39. Doshi JA, Takeshita J, Pinto L, et al. Biologic therapy adherence, discontinuation, switching, and restarting among patients with psoriasis in the US Medicare population. J Am Acad Dermatol. 2016;74(6):1057–1065.e4.

40. Ross C, Marshman G, Grillo M, Stanford T. Biological therapies for psoriasis: adherence and outcome analysis from a clinical perspective. Australas J Dermatol. 2016;57(2):137–40.

41. Strober MDPBE. Methotrexate and cyclosporine in psoriasis revisited. Semin Cutan Med Surg. 2014;33(2S):S27–30.

42. Gisondi P, Tessari G, Di Mercurio M, et al. Retention rate of systemic drugs in patients with chronic plaque psoriasis. Clin Dermatol. 2013;1(1):8–14.

43. Vidal D, Salleras M, Romani J, et al. Adherence of self-administered subcutaneous methotrexate in patients with chronic plaque-type psoriasis. J Eur Acad Dermatol Venereol. 2016;30(11):e131–2.

44. Dogra S, Yadav S. Acitretin in psoriasis: an evolving scenario. Int J Dermatol. 2014;53(5):525–38.

45. Shalom G, Cohen AD, Ziv M, et al. Biologic drug survival in Israeli psoriasis patients. J Am Acad Dermatol. 2017;76(4):662–669.e1.

46. Zhang P, Wu MX. A clinical review of phototherapy for psoriasis. Lasers Med Sci. 2018;33(1):173–80.
47. Racz E, Prens EP. Phototherapy of psoriasis, a chronic inflammatory skin disease. Adv Exp Med Biol. 2017;996:287–94.
48. Lynde CW, Gupta AK, Guenther L, Poulin Y, Levesque A, Bissonnette R. A randomized study comparing the combination of nbUVB and etanercept to etanercept monotherapy in patients with psoriasis who do not exhibit an excellent response after 12 weeks of etanercept. J Dermatolog Treat. 2012;23(4):261–7.
49. Nolan BV, Yentzer BA, Feldman SR. A review of home phototherapy for psoriasis. Dermatol Online J. 2010;16(2):1.
50. Thorneloe RJ, Bundy C, Griffiths CE, Ashcroft DM, Cordingley L. Nonadherence to psoriasis medication as an outcome of limited coping resources and conflicting goals: findings from a qualitative interview study with people with psoriasis. Br J Dermatol. 2017;176(3):667–76.
51. Feldman SR, Vrijens B, Gieler U, et al. Treatment adherence intervention studies in dermatology and guidance on how to support adherence. Am J Clin Dermatol. 2017;18(2):253–71.
52. Yelamos O, Ros S, Puig L. Improving patient outcomes in psoriasis: strategies to ensure treatment adherence. Psoriasis (Auckl). 2015;5:109–15.
53. Bewley A, Burrage DM, Ersser SJ, et al. Identifying individual psychosocial and adherence support needs in patients with psoriasis: a multinational two-stage qualitative and quantitative study. J Eur Acad Dermatol Venereol. 2014;28:763–70.
54. Ersser SJ, Cowdell FC, Latter SM, Healy E. Self-management experiences in adults with mild-moderate psoriasis: an exploratory study and implications for improved support. Br J Dermatol. 2010;163:1044–9.
55. D'Souza LS, Payette MJ. Estimated cost efficacy of systemic treatments that are approved by the US Food and Drug Administration for the treatment of moderate to severe psoriasis. J Am Acad Dermatol. 2015;72(4):589–98.
56. Lebwohl MG, Bachelez H, Barker J, et al. Patient perspectives in the management of psoriasis: results from the population-based Multinational Assessment of Psoriasis and Psoriatic Arthritis Survey. J Am Acad Dermatol. 2014;70(5):871–81.
57. Ros S, Puig L, Carrascosa JM. Cumulative life course impairment: the imprint of psoriasis on the patient's life. Actas Dermosifiliogr. 2014;105(2):128–34.
58. Aslam I, Feldman SR. Practical strategies to improve patient adherence to treatment regimens. South Med J. 2015;108:325–31.
59. Pouplard C, Gourraud PA, Meyer N, et al. Are we giving patients enough information on how to use topical treatments? Analysis of 767 prescriptions in psoriasis. Br J Dermatol. 2011;165:1332–6.
60. Martin SL, McGoey ST, Bebo BF Jr, Feldman SR. Patients' educational needs about topical treatments for psoriasis. J Am Acad Dermatol. 2013;68(6):e163–8.
61. Feldman SR. Approaching psoriasis differently: patient-physician relationships, patient education and choosing the right topical vehicle. J Drugs Dermatol. 2010;9:908–11.
62. Zirwas MJ, Holder JL. Patient education strategies in dermatology: Part 2: methods. J Clin Aesthet Dermatol. 2009;2:28–34.
63. Reich K, Zschocke I, Bachelez H, et al. A Topical Treatment Optimization Programme (TTOP) improves clinical outcome for calcipotriol/betamethasone gel in psoriasis: results of a 64-week multinational randomized phase IV study in 1790 patients (PSO-TOP). Br J Dermatol. 2017;177(1):197–205.
64. Caldarola G, De Simone C, Moretta G, Poscia A, Peris K. Role of personalized medication training in improving efficacy and adherence to a topical therapy in psoriatic patients. J Dermatolog Treat. 2017;28(8):722–5.
65. Bonnekoh B, Schmid-Ott G, Herold S, Sayegh-Jodehl S, Dierkes J, et al. Interdisciplinary training program for adults with psoriasis: six months follow-up. Hautarzt. 2006;57(10):917–22.
66. Wang W, Qiu Y, Zhao F, Zhang F. Poor medication adherence in patients with psoriasis and a successful intervention. J Dermatolog Treat. 2018;23:1–18.
67. Fenerty SD, West C, Davis SA, Kaplan SG, Feldman SR. The effect of reminder systems on patients' adherence to treatment. Patient Prefer Adherence. 2012;6:127–35.
68. Alpalhão M, Antunes J, Gouveia A, et al. A randomized controlled clinical trial to assess the impact of motivational phone calls on therapeutic adherence in patients suffering from psoriasis. Dermatol Ther. 2018;31(5):e12667.
69. Balato N, Megna M, Di Costanzo L, Balato A, Ayala F. Educational and motivational support service: a pilot study for mobile-phone-based interventions in patients with psoriasis. Br J Dermatol. 2013;168(1):201–5.
70. Svendsen MT, Andersen F, Andersen KH, et al. A smartphone application supporting patients with psoriasis improves adherence to topical treatment: a randomized controlled trial. Br J Dermatol. 2018;179(5):1062–71.
71. Umar N, Litaker D, Schaarschmidt ML, et al. Outcomes associated with matching patients' treatment preferences to physicians' recommendations: study methodology. BMC Health Serv Res. 2012;12:1–12.
72. Uhlenhake EE, Kurkowski D, Feldman SR. Conversations on psoriasis – what patients want and what physicians can provide: a qualitative look at patients and physician expectations. J Dermatolog Treat. 2010;21(1):6–12.
73. Zalewska A, Miniszewska J, Chodkiewicz J, Narbutt J. Acceptance of chronic illness in psoriasis vulgaris patients. J Eur Acad Dermatol Venereol. 2007;21(2):235–42.

74. Kulkarni AS, Balkrishnan R, Camacho FT, et al. Medication and health care service utilization related to depressive symptoms in older adults with psoriasis. J Drugs Dermatol. 2004;3:661–6.

75. Yentzer BA, Yelverton CB, Pearce DJ, Camacho FT, Makhzoumi Z, Clark A, et al. Adherence to acitretin and home narrowband ultraviolet B phototherapy in patients with psoriasis. J Am Acad Dermatol. 2008;59(4):577–81.

76. Koek MB, Buskens E, van Weelden H, Steegmans PH, Bruijnzeel-Koomen CA, Sigurdsson V. Home versus outpatient ultraviolet B phototherapy for mild to severe psoriasis: pragmatic multicentre randomised controlled non-inferiority trial (PLUTO study). BMJ. 2009;338:b1542.

77. Koek MB, Sigurdsson V, van Weelden H, Steegmans PH, Bruijnzeel-Koomen CA, Buskens E. Cost effectiveness of home ultraviolet B phototherapy for psoriasis: economic evaluation of a randomised controlled trial (PLUTO study). BMJ. 2010;340:c1490.

78. Cline A, Unrue EL, Collins A, Feldman SR. Adherence to a novel home phototherapy system with integrated features. Dermatol Online J. 2019;25(3):3.

Chapter 8
Adherence in Atopic Dermatitis

Sree S. Kolli, Adrian Pona, Abigail Cline, Lindsay C. Strowd, and Steven R. Feldman

Introduction

Atopic dermatitis (AD) is a chronic inflammatory skin disease that begins early in childhood and persists until adulthood. AD affects up to 11% of children in the United States and 20% worldwide [1, 2]. With impacts on sleep and social and intellectual development, AD can cause children and families to have a diminished quality of life. AD is a multibillion dollar problem to society, with an estimated direct cost of $900 million per year in the United States [3].

Management involves a variety of topical therapies including topical corticosteroids (TCS), topical calcineurin inhibitors (TCI), and emollients. When topical therapies fail, phototherapy and systemic treatments are initiated. Phototherapy can be an inconvenient option, whereas systemic treatment with prednisone, methotrexate, or cyclosporine can have long-term toxicity. Combating the burden of this disease requires a sophisticated approach, but treatment plans often compromise adherence to treatment. About 30% of AD patients do not take their medications as prescribed [4]. Research on the factors that affect patients' adherence to treatment also has the potential to vastly improve patients' outcomes and to do so quickly and at low cost. Nonadherence can be due to primary nonadherence, where patients fail to redeem their prescriptions, or secondary nonadherence, where patients do not take their medication as directed. This chapter will look at the prevalence of nonadherence in AD patients, barriers to adherence, and potential interventions for this subset of patients.

S. S. Kolli (✉) · A. Pona · A. Cline
Department of Dermatology, Wake Forest School of Medicine, Winston-Salem, NC, USA
e-mail: skolli@wakehealth.edu

L. C. Strowd
Center for Dermatology Research, Department of Dermatology, Wake Forest School of Medicine, Winston-Salem, NC, USA

S. R. Feldman
Departments of Dermatology, Pathology and Social Sciences & Health Policy, Wake Forest School of Medicine, Winston-Salem, NC, USA

© Springer Nature Switzerland AG 2020
S. R. Feldman et al. (eds.), *Treatment Adherence in Dermatology*, Updates in Clinical Dermatology, https://doi.org/10.1007/978-3-030-27809-0_8

Prevalence of Nonadherence in Atopic Dermatitis

Numerous studies have assessed adherence rates in AD. A study assessed primary nonadherence in 322 subjects at an outpatient dermatology clinic. They analyzed the frequency of prescriptions filled within 4 weeks of their appointment. Of 137 AD subjects given a new prescription, 31.4% did not redeem their prescriptions [5].

Once patients fill their prescriptions, many patients still do not take their medication as directed. In one study, only 50% of patients initiated treatment during an acute AD flare with an average treatment delay of 7 days [6]. For long-term management of AD, many patients fail to use the proper amount of medication. Patients may underuse or overuse medications leading to insufficient treatment response. In a study evaluating the efficacy of a topical tacrolimus in adult AD subjects, 66.7% underused the prescribed medication, 12.4% overused, and 20.9% used the proper amount [7]. Those who underused the recommended treatment reported poorer improvement in Eczema Area and Severity Index (EASI) score than those who used the proper amount of medication (1.64 vs 4.65) [7].

Despite high self-reports of adherence by patients, the adherence rate as measured by electronic monitoring is far from perfect. Of 25 AD patients using twice daily hydrocortisone 17-butyrate 0.1% in one of three vehicles, 70% adhered to the medication despite nearly all patients self-reporting perfect usage of the medication [8]. Another study involved 41 subjects with mild-to-moderate AD who were instructed to use desonide hydrogel 0.05% twice daily. Mean adherence declined over time from 81% on day 1 to 50% by Day 27 [9]. Although self-reported adherence rate was 87% among AD subjects using clocortolone pivalate cream 0.1% at Week 4, the average adherence rate determined by electronic monitoring was 70% [10].

Even short-term treatment results in poor adherence. When 10 subjects with mild-to-moderate AD were instructed to apply fluocinonide cream 0.1% twice daily for 5 days, the mean adherence rate measured by electronic monitoring was 40% [11].

There is a high prevalence of nonadherence in AD as assessed by clinical trials evidence. Furthermore, adherence rates are often overestimated in clinical trials so there is concern that adherence is much poorer in clinical practice. Poor adherence may explain suboptimal treatment response and therefore should recognized and addressed before switching to a more harmful medication.

Nonadherence Goes Beyond Topical Corticosteroids

Topical corticosteroids are first-line treatments for AD. Much of the data on adherence comes from the use of these topical agents; however, there are a variety of other topical therapies that are used in AD that may also present challenges to adherence. These include moisturizers, wet-wrap therapy, topical calcineurin inhibitors, and topical phosphodiesterase 4 inhibitors.

Moisturizers

Daily moisturizer use is standard of care treatment for AD prevention and maintenance therapy [12]. Moisturizers include emollients, humectants, and occlusive agents. Nonadherence may be an issue if these agents misalign with patient preference and cause inconvenience. The most commonly cited reasons for nonadherence to moisturizers are skin discomfort (27%), time-consuming application (22%), and cost (23%) [13]. Although providers prefer creams and ointment moisturizer vehicles due to their effectiveness, their thicker consistency, in contrast to lotions, may impede adherence. Occlusive agents are very greasy, have a strong odor, contain potential allergens, and cause folliculitis when inappropriately used [14]. AD patients prefer a moisturizer based on "consistency," whether it "absorbs fast," and is "nice to wear." [15].

In addition to inconvenient moisturizer application, 23% of AD patients believe that moisturizers play a minimal role in managing eczema [13]. About 75% of AD caregivers believe emollients provide short-term relief but there are barriers for long-term use [16]. Some caregivers believe emollients are "unnatural," contain "chemicals," and the skin gets "used to emollients" thus losing effectiveness with regular use [16]. Patient belief is a large barrier to nonadherence. Although most caregivers agree emollients help with active disease, some reported mixed feelings when using emollients during disease remission [16].

Wet-Wrap Therapy

Wet-wrap therapy is indicated for severe or refractory AD [12]. Wet-wrap therapy consists of a wet layer of occlusive bandages followed by dryer outer layer. Wet-wrap therapy increases contact time with topical therapies resulting in increased absorption. Due to its messiness, inconvenience, feasibility, and time-consuming application, it may be a less attractive option for children and caregivers. Other common adherence barriers to wet-wrap therapy include high cost, special training in usage, unpleasant sensation of cold damp wraps, increased risk of cutaneous infection, and poor tolerability [17].

Topical Calcineurin Inhibitors

Topical calcineurin inhibitors (TCIs) are second-line therapies, appropriate for thin and sensitive skin that may not tolerate TCS. TCIs include tacrolimus ointment (0.03% for patients over 2 years and 0.1% for patients >15 years) and pimecrolimus cream (1% for patients >2 years) [12]. Tacrolimus is Food and Drug Administration (FDA)-approved for moderate-to-severe AD whereas pimecrolimus is approved for mild-to-moderate AD. Common side effects of TCIs include burning and stinging; the label contains a black box warning for potential malignancy. The black box warning may raise concerns that impede patient adherence, even though there is considerable evidence that topical calcineurin inhibitors do not cause an increased risk of cancer. A study assessed adherence in 200 AD patients who were instructed to apply topical tacrolimus twice daily; the average number of applications per day was 1.75 ± 0.53 and there was a steep decline in adherence from the first to second week (73.5% vs 61%) [18].

Topical Phosphodiesterase 4 Inhibitors

Crisaborole has been recently FDA-approved for mild-to-moderate AD in patients 2 years and older. Although crisaborole does not have the adverse effect profile of topical corticosteroids, application site pain is a common finding that may impede adherence [19]. Other reasons for nonadherence include high cost and slow onset of action.

Barriers to Adherence

Many barriers impact adherence in AD ranging from poor education, beliefs, inconvenience, poor patient-physician relationship, forgetfulness, poor accountability, and cost (Fig. 8.1) [20, 21].

Knowledge Gaps and Fears of Adverse Effects

Often, patients may not be fully aware of the benefits of moisturizers and adjunctive therapies such as TCI in managing AD and fear the risks of TCS [22]. In a survey of caregivers with children suffering from dermatological conditions, the most commonly cited concern about medication use was a fear of side effects [23]. Of 208 AD patients, 80.7% reported fear of TCS. There was a positive correlation between the fear of TCS and the belief that topical corticosteroids pass through the skin into the bloodstream (B-coefficient = 0.63, $P < 0.001$), inconsistent information about the quantity of cream to apply (B-coefficient = 0.34, $P < 0.05$), and poor treatment adherence (B-coefficient = 0.53, $P < 0.05$) [24]. Of 77 caregivers, 64% reported that they worry a lot about using topical corticosteroids on their child. Caregivers most frequently worry over skin atrophy [25].

Poor Communication

Poor communication and misalignment with patients' preferences are common impediments to adherence. Patients may be confused about the different potencies of TCS and how to appropriately apply the medication [26]. In a survey identifying reasons for nonadherence to topical therapies, 18.2% reported unclear instructions as a common barrier to optimal management [27]. With complex treatment regimens, only 24% of AD caregivers feel confident they can manage AD flares and 75% felt that the most important determinant in their child's quality of life was effectively controlling their AD [6].

Patients may prefer some types of treatments over others in order to minimize inconvenience arising from messy application, strong odor, and time-consuming regimens [22]. Patients may also prefer a particular type of vehicle in regards to topical corticosteroids and moisturizers [9, 28].

Forgetfulness

Forgetfulness is a common cause of unintentional nonadherence, especially in chronic diseases like AD. About 80% of nonadherent subjects attribute poor adherence to forgetfulness [27]. To address forgetfulness, incorporating required medications into an existing daily routine may help. One approach might be to apply the medication every morning after breakfast [29]. Pediatric AD patients may benefit from sticker calendar charts. A sticker is placed on each day of the calendar following appropriate use of the medication providing positive reinforcement and a reminder for the next dose [30].

Adherence Interventions for Atopic Dermatitis

To overcome such barriers, interventions including educational workshops, written action plans, reminder devices, early follow-up visits, and substituting for affordable generic medications may improve adherence (Table 8.1).

Education Workshops

In order to improve understanding of AD treatments and reduce fears, educational workshops may be effective tools in improving patient and caregiver knowledge about the disease and therapies, provide hands-on training in medication application and address any questions or concerns about adverse

Fig. 8.1 Overcoming barriers to nonadherence [20, 21]

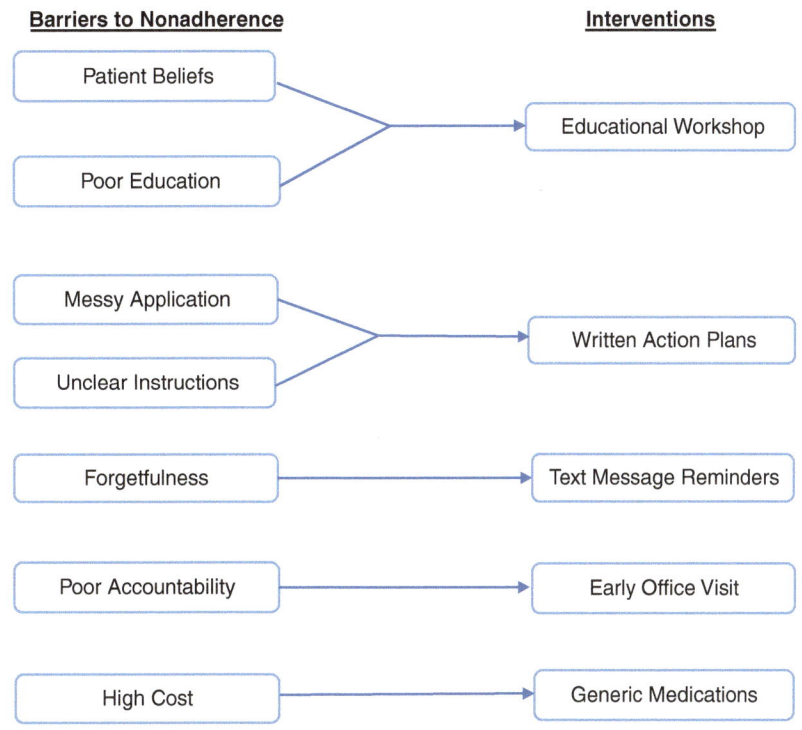

effects. Educational workshops provide personalized, in-person training to help empower patients and caregivers to manage AD.

A randomized control trial (RCT) of 61 pediatric subjects evaluated the effectiveness of a 2-hour educational workshop constituting lectures about AD, management, and hands-on training in wet-wrap therapy and topical application. During follow-up visits, disease severity was assessed using the Scoring of Atopic Dermatitis index (SCORAD) and quality of life using the Infant Dermatology Quality of Life Index (IDQLI). Improved disease severity served as a measure of adherence. The intervention group resulted in greater improvement in disease severity compared to control (53.9% vs 15.8%, $P < 0.05$). There was no difference in quality of life between groups ($P > 0.05$) [31]. Another type of educational workshop led to promising results. A RCT of 99 AD subjects were stratified to a specialized nurse-led educational workshop or a dermatologist-led workshop. The nurse-led workshop was 90 minutes while the dermatologist-led workshop was 40 minutes. AD severity was measured using SCORAD. After 4 weeks, the nurse-led workshop resulted in a 9.93-point improvement in SCORAD compared to dermatologist led-group ($P < 0.001$). About 73% in the nurse-led group improved to mild eczema compared to 40% in dermatologist-led group. Subjects in the nurse-led workshop group bathed more often (29%), applied emollients more frequently (80%), and used wet-wrap therapy more often (76%) compared to the dermatologist-led group (8%, 62%, and 12%, respectively) at the follow-up visit. In addition, 34% in the dermatologist-led group used TCS improperly compared to 8% in nurse-led group [32].

AD patients may benefit from attending multiple educational workshops. A study randomized 204 AD subjects to six 2-hour educational workshops or standard care. The six sessions took an interdisciplinary approach involving pediatricians, psychologists, and nutritionists. At a 1-year follow-up, 82% in the intervention group used regular skin care products including topical corticosteroids and emollients compared to 67% in the control group ($P = 0.041$). About 65% in intervention group used topical corticosteroids compared to 38% in control group ($P = 0.001$). In addition, the intervention

Table 8.1 Interventions for improving adherence in atopic dermatitis patients

Author	Study design	Intervention	Number of subjects	Primary outcome	Result
Educational workshops					
Grillo et al. [31]	RCT	2-hour educational workshop	61	SCORAD	Intervention:53.9% vs control: 15.8%; $P < 0.05$
				IDQLI, CDLQI, DFI	No difference between groups
Moore et al. [32]	RCT	Nurse-led educational workshop	99	SCORAD	Intervention: 73% vs control: 40%; $P < 0.001$
Staab et al. [33]	RCT	6 sessions of 2-hr educational workshops	204	SCORAD	No significant difference between groups; $P = 0.43$
				Treatment habits-use of TCS	Intervention: 65% vs control: 38%; $P = 0.041$
Shaw et al. [34]	RCT	15-minute educational workshop	106	SCORAD	No significant difference between groups
				IDQLI	No significant difference between groups
Chinn et al. [35]	RCT	30-minute educational workshop	235	IDQLI	No significant difference between groups
Written action plan					
Rork et al. [37]	Non-RCT	EAP	35	Telephone survey 3–12 months later assessing disease severity and helpfulness of EAP	68% of children improved from baseline and 86% found EAP helpful
Gilliam et al. [38]	RCT	EAP	88	Childhood AD impact score-quality of life	No significant difference between groups
Text messaging					
Pena-Robichaux et al. [40]	Non-RCT	Daily text message reminders	25	Self-reported medication diary and self-reported forgetfulness in taking medication	72% improvement in adherence compared to baseline; $P < 0.001$
Singer et al. [41]	RCT	Daily text message reminder	30	EASI	Intervention: 58% vs control:53%; $P > 0.05$
				AD knowledge quiz	Intervention:84.6% vs control: 74.8%; $P = 0.04$
Early follow-up					
Sagransky et al. [43]	RCT	Early 1-week follow-up	20	Medication event monitoring system-adherence	Intervention:69% vs control: 54%; $P > 0.05$
				EASI	Intervention: 76% vs control: 45%; $P > 0.05$

SCORAD Scoring of Atopic Dermatitis index, *IDQLI* Infant Dermatology Quality of Life Index, *CDLQI* Children Dermatology Life Quality Index, *DFI* Dermatitis Family Impact, *EASI* Eczema Area and Severity Index, *RCT* Randomized Control Trial, *EAP* Eczema Action Plan resulted in reduced treatment costs at 1-year follow-up compared to control (119 vs 65 euros $P = 0.043$) suggesting better self-management and reduced healthcare use [33].

Another RCT assessed the effectiveness of a 15-minute individualized educational session in improving disease severity and quality of life in 106 AD pediatric subjects. The educational session involved training in the proper use of topical therapies, bathing habits, and an opportunity to address concerns. There was no difference in SCORAD or quality of life measures between both groups [34]. A similar RCT assessed the effectiveness of a 30-minute educational workshop on quality of life in 235 pediatric AD subjects. The intervention involved a demonstration of topical medication application along with advice and education by a dermatology nurse. Patients were provided one-page educational leaflets. There was no difference in quality of life between groups at 4 or 12-week follow-up visits [35].

Multiple, time-intensive educational workshops seem most helpful in improving adherence in AD. Workshops provide opportunities to train and educate patients on topical application, hands-on training, and improved understanding of topical therapy efficacy and potentially reducing fears about adverse effects. Patients may become more willing to initiate and maintain the recommended treatment regimen.

Written Action Plans

Written action plans, also known as Eczema Action Plans (EAPs), are effective tools that provide clear instructions and incorporate patients' preferences. EAPs may be helpful for developing a trusting patient-provider relationship, as these action plans involve patients in developing a treatment regimen and thus strengthening patient adherence.

Many AD patients and providers believe EAPs are beneficial in improving self-management. About 79% of pediatric dermatologists endorse EAPs as a means to improve adherence [36]. The effectiveness of EAPs on disease severity was measured by a self-reported survey of 35 AD caregivers. About 86% of caregivers found EAPs helpful in managing AD flares and 68% associated them with disease improvement [37]. A RCT evaluating the use of EAP among 88 AD subjects resulted in improved the quality of life ($P = 0.004$) and symptomatology ($P = 0.040$) compared to baseline. However, there was no difference between intervention and control group [38].

Reminders

Text message reminders have recently been used as a novel technique to improve adherence. A 6-week pilot study assessed the effectiveness of daily text message [39] reminders on adherence of 25 AD subjects. Subjects completed a self-reported medication diary and survey of how often they forgot to use their medication. About 72% of participants improved in adherence in both aforementioned measures compared to baseline ($P < 0.001$) at Week 6. About 88% found TM reminders helpful and 84% would continue with TM reminders. Around 72% said that they would be willing to pay a small monthly fee for the service [40]. A RCT assessed the effectiveness of daily TM reminders in 30 AD subjects. Disease severity was measured using the EASI and an AD knowledge quiz was administered. The intervention group has a greater improvement in EASI compared to control, although the difference was not statistically significant (58% vs 53%, $P > 0.05$). Quiz scores were higher in the intervention group compared to control (84.6% vs 74.8%, $P = 0.04$) [41].

Improving Accountability

Medication adherence often increases around the time of follow-up visits due to "white coat compliance." [42] Introducing early and frequent follow-up visits after implementing a new AD treatment regimen increases the likelihood of prescription redemption and medication use. This may lead to earlier treatment response and greater long-term adherence as AD patients are more likely to continue taking their medications once they experience improvement. A RCT assessed the effectiveness of an extra office visit in 30 AD subjects instructed to apply tacrolimus ointment 0.03% twice daily. Patients in the intervention group followed up at Weeks 1 and 4 while the control group followed up at Week 4. Adherence was measured by Medication Event Monitoring System caps. The intervention group had a higher mean adherence rate compared to control (69% vs 54%, respectively, $P > 0.05$) and greater EASI improvement (76% vs 45%, respectively, $P > 0.05$) [43]. A small sample size may have contributed to a lack of statistically significance between groups.

Combating High Medication Cost

High cost associated with AD medications and care is an important and often overlooked reason for nonadherence [23]. There has been an increase in Medicare and out-of-pocket spending on topical steroids in part due to the higher costs of medication. Medicare Part D expenditures on topical steroids between 2011 and 2015 was 2.3 billion dollars whereas out-of-pocket spending was 333.7 million dollars during the same time period [44].

A potential solution is using electronic medical record support tools that enable substitution for the most affordable generic topical steroid [44]. There are also financial resources available for AD patients including NeedyMeds, Rx outreach, and PAN foundation that can be offered for patients during clinic visits. In addition, promoting adherence leads to disease control and long-term cost-effectiveness.

Conclusion

AD requires long-term management with topical therapies. Nonadherence is prevalent among AD populations due to steroid phobia, inconvenience, and high cost. Helpful interventions include educational workshops, EAPs, TM reminders, and early and frequent follow-up visits. Promoting adherence in AD leads to better treatment outcomes, economic burden, and quality of life.

Funding sources None

Conflicts of Interest Feldman has received research, speaking and/or consulting support from a variety of companies including Galderma, GSK/Stiefel, Almirall, Leo Pharma, Boehringer Ingelheim, Mylan, Celgene, Pfizer, Valeant, Abbvie, Samsung, Janssen, Lilly, Menlo, Merck, Novartis, Regeneron, Sanofi, Novan, Qurient, National Biological Corporation, Caremark, Advance Medical, Sun Pharma, Suncare Research, Informa, UpToDate and National Psoriasis Foundation. He is founder and majority owner of www.DrScore.com and founder and part owner of Causa Research, a company dedicated to enhancing patients' adherence to treatment. Dr. Lindsay Strowd has received grant support from Pfizer, consulting support from Sandofi Regeneron Granzyme and is a speaker for Actelion.

Sree Kolli, Adrian Pona and Abigail Cline have no conflicts to disclose.

References

1. Williams H, Robertson C, Stewart A, Ait-Khaled N, Anabwani G, Anderson R, et al. Worldwide variations in the prevalence of symptoms of atopic eczema in the International Study of Asthma and Allergies in Childhood. J Allergy Clin Immunol. 1999;103(1. Pt 1):125–38.
2. Shaw TE, Currie GP, Koudelka CW, Simpson EL. Eczema prevalence in the United States: data from the 2003 National Survey of Children's Health. J Invest Dermatol. 2011;131(1):67–73.
3. Su JC, Kemp AS, Varigos GA, Nolan TM. Atopic eczema: its impact on the family and financial cost. Arch Dis Child. 1997;76(2):159–62.
4. Krejci-Manwaring J, Tusa MG, Carroll C, Camacho F, Kaur M, Carr D, et al. Stealth monitoring of adherence to topical medication: adherence is very poor in children with atopic dermatitis. J Am Acad Dermatol. 2007;56(2):211–6.
5. Storm A, Andersen SE, Benfeldt E, Serup J. One in 3 prescriptions are never redeemed: primary nonadherence in an outpatient clinic. J Am Acad Dermatol. 2008;59(1):27–33.
6. Zuberbier T, Orlow SJ, Paller AS, Taieb A, Allen R, Hernanz-Hermosa JM, et al. Patient perspectives on the management of atopic dermatitis. J Allergy Clin Immunol. 2006;118(1):226–32.
7. Yang MY, Jin H, Shim WH, Kim GW, Kim HS, Ko HC, et al. High rates of secondary non-adherence causes decreased efficacy of 0.1% topical tacrolimus in adult eczema patients: results from a multicenter clinical trial. J Dermatolog Treat. 2018;29(2):129–34.
8. Wilson R, Camacho F, Clark AR, Young T, Inabinet R, Yentzer BA, et al. Adherence to topical hydrocortisone 17-butyrate 0.1% in different vehicles in adults with atopic dermatitis. J Am Acad Dermatol. 2009;60(1):166–8.
9. Yentzer BA, Camacho FT, Young T, Fountain JM, Clark AR, Feldman SR. Good adherence and early efficacy using desonide hydrogel for atopic dermatitis: results from a program addressing patient compliance. J Drugs Dermatol. 2010;9(4):324–9.
10. Conde JF, Kaur M, Fleischer AB Jr, Tusa MG, Camacho F, Feldman SR. Adherence to clocortolone pivalate cream 0.1% in a pediatric population with atopic dermatitis. Cutis. 2008;81(5):435–41.
11. Hix E, Gustafson CJ, O'Neill JL, Huang K, Sandoval LF, Harrison J, et al. Adherence to a five day treatment course of topical fluocinonide 0.1% cream in atopic dermatitis. Dermatol Online J. 2013;19(10):20029.
12. Fleischer DM, Udkoff J, Borok J, Friedman A, Nicol N, Bienstock J, et al. Atopic dermatitis: skin care and topical therapies. Semin Cutan Med Surg. 2017;36(3):104–10.
13. Huynh RK, Wong HH, Aw D, Toh M. Adherence to topical corticosteroids and moisturisers in adults with endogenous eczema in Singapore. Hong Kong J Dermatol Venereol. 2015;23:161–74.
14. Kraft JN, Lynde CW. Moisturizers: what they are and a practical approach to product selection. Skin Therapy Lett. 2005;10(5):1–8.
15. Joergensen KM, Jemec GBE. Use of moisturizers among Danish atopic dermatitis patients-which perceived product characteristics associate with long-term adherence? J Dermatolog Treat. 2018;29(2):116–22.
16. Santer M, Muller I, Yardley L, Lewis-Jones S, Ersser S, Little P. Parents' and carers' views about emollients for childhood eczema: qualitative interview study. BMJ open. 2016;6(8):e011887.
17. Oranje AP, Devillers AC, Kunz B, Jones SL, DeRaeve L, Van Gysel D, et al. Treatment of patients with atopic dermatitis using wet-wrap dressings with diluted steroids and/or emollients. An expert panel's opinion and review of the literature. J Eur Acad Dermatol Venereol. 2006;20(10):1277–86.
18. Jin H, Kim JM, Kim GW, Kim HS, Ko HC, Kim MB, et al. Inappropriate amounts of topical tacrolimus applied on Korean patients with eczema. J Dermatolog Treat. 2017;28(4):327–31.
19. Lin CP, Gordon S, Her MJ, Rosmarin D. A retrospective study: application site pain with the use of crisaborole, a topical PDE4 inhibitor. J Am Acad Dermatol. 2018;80(5):1451–3.
20. Brown KK, Rehmus WE, Kimball AB. Determining the relative importance of patient motivations for nonadherence to topical corticosteroid therapy in psoriasis. J Am Acad Dermatol. 2006;55(4):607–13.
21. Feldman SR, Vrijens B, Gieler U, Piaserico S, Puig L, van de Kerkhof P. Treatment adherence intervention studies in dermatology and guidance on how to support adherence. Am J Clin Dermatol. 2017;18(2):253–71.
22. Fouere S, Adjadj L, Pawin H. How patients experience psoriasis: results from a European survey. J Eur Acad Dermatol Venereol. 2005;19(Suppl 3):2–6.
23. Ellis RM, Koch LH, McGuire E, Williams JV. Potential barriers to adherence in pediatric dermatology. Pediatr Dermatol. 2011;28(3):242–4.
24. Aubert-Wastiaux H, Moret L, Le Rhun A, Fontenoy AM, Nguyen JM, Leux C, et al. Topical corticosteroid phobia in atopic dermatitis: a study of its nature, origins and frequency. Br J Dermatol. 2011;165(4):808–14.
25. Gustavsen HE, Gjersvik P. Topical corticosteroid phobia among parents of children with atopic dermatitis in a semirural area of Norway. J Eur Acad Dermatol Venereol. 2016;30(1):168.
26. Savary J, Ortonne JP, Aractingi S. The right dose in the right place: an overview of current prescription, instruction and application modalities for topical psoriasis treatments. J Eur Acad Dermatol Venereol. 2005;19(Suppl 3):14–7.

27. Choi JW, Kim BR, Youn SW. Adherence to topical therapies for the treatment of psoriasis: surveys of physicians and patients. Ann Dermatol. 2017;29(5):559–64.

28. Fenerty SD, O'Neill JL, Gustafson CJ, Feldman SR. Maternal adherence factors in the treatment of pediatric atopic dermatitis. JAMA Dermatol. 2013;149(2):229–31.

29. Santer M, Burgess H, Yardley L, Ersser SJ, Lewis-Jones S, Muller I, et al. Managing childhood eczema: qualitative study exploring carers' experiences of barriers and facilitators to treatment adherence. J Adv Nurs. 2013;69(11):2493–501.

30. Luersen K, Davis SA, Kaplan SG, Abel TD, Winchester WW, Feldman SR. Sticker charts: a method for improving adherence to treatment of chronic diseases in children. Pediatr Dermatol. 2012;29(4):403–8.

31. Grillo M, Gassner L, Marshman G, Dunn S, Hudson P. Pediatric atopic eczema: the impact of an educational intervention. Pediatr Dermatol. 2006;23(5):428–36.

32. Moore EJ, Williams A, Manias E, Varigos G, Donath S. Eczema workshops reduce severity of childhood atopic eczema. Australas J Dermatol. 2009;50(2):100–6.

33. Staab D, von Rueden U, Kehrt R, Erhart M, Wenninger K, Kamtsiuris P, et al. Evaluation of a parental training program for the management of childhood atopic dermatitis. Pediatr Allergy Immunol. 2002;13(2):84–90.

34. Shaw M, Morrell DS, Goldsmith LA. A study of targeted enhanced patient care for pediatric atopic dermatitis (STEP PAD). Pediatr Dermatol. 2008;25(1):19–24.

35. Chinn DJ, Poyner T, Sibley G. Randomized controlled trial of a single dermatology nurse consultation in primary care on the quality of life of children with atopic eczema. Br J Dermatol. 2002;146(3):432–9.

36. Stringer T, Yin HS, Oza VS. A survey to assess use patterns and perceptions of efficacy of eczema action plans among pediatric dermatologists. Pediatr Dermatol. 2018;35(6):e432–e4.

37. Rork JF, Sheehan WJ, Gaffin JM, Timmons KG, Sidbury R, Schneider LC, et al. Parental response to written eczema action plans in children with eczema. Arch Dermatol. 2012;148(3):391–2.

38. Gilliam AE, Madden N, Sendowski M, Mioduszewski M, Duderstadt KG. Use of Eczema Action Plans (EAPs) to improve parental understanding of treatment regimens in pediatric atopic dermatitis (AD): a randomized controlled trial. J Am Acad Dermatol. 2016;74(2):375–7.e1-3.

39. Lee E, Trepicchio WL, Oestreicher JL, Pittman D, Wang F, Chamian F, et al. Increased expression of interleukin 23 p19 and p40 in lesional skin of patients with psoriasis vulgaris. J Exp Med. 2004;199(1):125–30.

40. Pena-Robichaux V, Kvedar JC, Watson AJ. Text messages as a reminder aid and educational tool in adults and adolescents with atopic dermatitis: a pilot study. Dermatol Res Pract. 2010;2010:894258.

41. Singer HM, Levin LE, Morel KD, Garzon MC, Stockwell MS, Lauren CT. Texting atopic dermatitis patients to optimize learning and eczema area and severity index scores: a pilot randomized control trial. Pediatr Dermatol. 2018;35(4):453–7.

42. Feldman SR, Camacho FT, Krejci-Manwaring J, Carroll CL, Balkrishnan R. Adherence to topical therapy increases around the time of office visits. J Am Acad Dermatol. 2007;57(1):81–3.

43. Sagransky MJ, Yentzer BA, Williams LL, Clark AR, Taylor SL, Feldman SR. A randomized controlled pilot study of the effects of an extra office visit on adherence and outcomes in atopic dermatitis. Arch Dermatol. 2010;146(12):1428–30.

44. Song H, Adamson A, Mostaghimi A. Medicare Part D payments for topical steroids: rising costs and potential savings. JAMA Dermatol. 2017;153(8):755–9.

Chapter 9
Adherence in Acne

Wasim Haidari, Katelyn R. Glines, Abigail Cline, and Steven R. Feldman

Introduction

Acne vulgaris is chronic inflammatory skin disorder with complex pathogenesis [1]. Disease pathophysiology is multifactorial with hyperseborrhea and dyseborrhea, altered keratinization of the sebaceous duct, *Cutibacterium acnes (C. acnes)* colonization, and inflammation all playing an important role [1]. Hormones contributing to the development of acne include androgens, insulins, and insulin-like growth factor-1. Adding to the complexity are alterations in sebum production, hypersensitivity to androgen production, and inflammatory cytokines affected by the innate immune system. Targeting the various pathogenic factors is one of the general principles of acne treatment, and is the reason why multiple acne treatments exist [2]. Treatment of acne is complex, ranging from various topical to oral agents, and more recently new devices and laser treatments [2].

Acne affects more than 85% of teenagers and the disease may continue into adulthood. While not life threatening, acne is linked with negative impact on quality of life (QOL) and self esteem [3]. Various factors such as one's ethnic background, personality, sex, age, severity of disease, and presence of scarring determine the impact on QOL. In a recent cross-sectional, case-control study assessing QOL and self-esteem in 100 acne patients, 58% of the cases had medium-to-high impairment in QOL according Cardiff Acne Disability Index (CADI). This study also identified that the QOL impairment worsens as disease severity increases [4]. Nevertheless, while acne can have a major impact on QOL, patients still may not use recommended treatment.

Adherence to even simple acne regimens is poor; adherence to more complex regimens is worse [5]. Low adherence to treatment in the adolescent population is highly prevalent. Special approaches may be needed in this patient population to promote good adherence to treatment. This chapter will

W. Haidari (✉) · K. R. Glines
Center for Dermatology Research, Department of Dermatology,
Wake Forest School of Medicine, Winston-Salem, NC, USA
e-mail: whaidari@wakehealth.edu

A. Cline
Department of Dermatology, Wake Forest School of Medicine, Winston-Salem, NC, USA

S. R. Feldman
Departments of Dermatology, Pathology and Social Sciences & Health Policy, Wake Forest School of Medicine, Winston-Salem, NC, USA

© Springer Nature Switzerland AG 2020   85
S. R. Feldman et al. (eds.), *Treatment Adherence in Dermatology*, Updates in Clinical Dermatology,
https://doi.org/10.1007/978-3-030-27809-0_9

evaluate the prevalence of nonadherence in acne, analyze nonadherence among different acne treatments, and discuss interventions to improve adherence.

Prevalence of Nonadherence in Acne

As medication adherence is very important to the success of acne treatment, numerous studies have evaluated adherence rates in acne patients (Table 9.1). Acne patients have high rates of primary nonadherence, which is the failure to procure and initiate a prescribed medication [6]. Twenty-seven percent of acne medication prescriptions were not started in the first 3 months. Thirty-four percent of prescriptions go unfilled by 3 months; however, when patients were surveyed why they failed to pick up their prescriptions, only 6% admitted to primary nonadherence [6].

Filling the prescription is only the first step. Patients still need take their medications as directed by a healthcare provider. Secondary nonadherence refers to patients not using their prescriptions as instructed, missing doses, or discontinuing therapy early. In a survey of 428 acne patients, 76% of subjects reported poor adherence. Adherence to topical medication was poor in 52% of those treated with a topical agent only (n = 123), and in 49% of subjected taking combination therapies (n = 275). Patients who reported a good understanding of acne and its treatment were more likely to have good adherence [7].

In a retrospective cohort study evaluating acne medication adherence in 24,438 patients Medicacid patients, of whom 89% were under the age of 18, *only 12% of the patients were adherent!* Patient's age, gender, number of drug refills and number of drug classes used are the main factors associated with adherence [8]. In children and adolescent Medicaid patients with acne, only 4% of children and 13% of adolescents were adherent [9].

Other issues with adherence to acne treatments which can all lead to treatment failure, include adherence decreasing over time, drug holidays in which patients go several days or more without taking medication, misunderstanding how the medication is supposed to be used, and overusing

Table 9.1 Prevalence of nonadherence in acne patients

Study	Sample size	Measure of adherence	Key results
Miyachi et al. [7]	N = 428	Self-reported	76% of subjects reported poor adherence. Adherence to topical medication was poor in 52% of those treated with a topical agent (N = 123), and in 49% of subjects taking combination therapies (N = 275).
Hester et al. [9]	N = 24,438	The adherence rate was measured using MPR; the MPR was dichotomized to categorize patients as adherent (≥0.8) or nonadherent (<0.8)	89% of subjects were under the age 18. *Only 12% of the patients were adherent!* In children and adolescent medicaid patients with acne, only 4% of children and 13% of adolescents were adherent.
Huyler et al. [16]	N = 84	Self-reported	Among the 84 patients recommneded OTC benzoyl peroxide by their physician, only 36% of patients included an OTC recommendation when recounting treatment plan verbally.
Biset et al. [52]	N = 67,657	Adherence was measured according to the MPR; patients were considered adherent if MPR was ≥0.8	46.1% of patients receiving isotretinoin had MPR ≥ 0.8. This percentage decreased as the number of attempts increased (29.8% for the second attempt and 19.8% for more than two attempts).

MPR Medication Possession Ratio, *OTC* Over-the-counter

medications. A study analyzing data from MarketScan database differentiated acne treatment adherence to specific medication classes. Oral therapies (retinoids, 57%; antibiotics, 4%; contraceptives, 49%, glucocorticoids: 2%) had better adherence than topical formulations (retinoids, 2%; antibiotics, 4%; and glucocorticoids, 2%) [10]. Better adherence to treatment regimens results in improved clinical outcomes. To address the insufficient treatment response of acne patients, it is worthwhile to evaluate patient adherence before switching treatments or adding to the complexity of the patient's treatment.

Nonadherence to Topical Therapy

Topical Retinoids

First generation all-trans retinoic acid (tretinoin) and third-generation (adapalene and tazarotene) topical retinoids serve as the cornerstone for treatment of comedonal and inflammatory acne [2]. Retinoids are anti-inflammatory, comedolytic, and resolve the precursor lesion. These medications enhance any topical acne regimen and are ideal for comedonal acne [11]. In the study of Japanese patients with acne, topical retinoids were prescribed in 47% of the patients, with a higher likelihood of use in males (54% vs 44%, respectively); however, the use of topical retinoids increased with increasing severity of acne (40% with mild acne to 52% with severe acne) [7].

Common reasons for premature discontinuation of retinoids are irritation with initial use of medication, lag time until patients see improvement, and the complexity of treatment regimens [12]. In addition to taking some time to work, the disadvantage of topical therapy is that it can be laborious and time-consuming for patients [13].

Topical Antibiotics

Commonly prescribed topical antibacterial agents include clindamycin, erythromycin, and dapsone. Clindamycin and erythromycin provide coverage against *Staphylococcus aureus* and *C. acnes* [2]. These agents are effective first-line treatments for mild-to-moderate acne, but are not recommended as monotherapy due do the risk of developing antibiotic resistance. They are commonly prescribed with benzoyl peroxide to decrease this risk. Adverse effects of clindamycin and erythromycin may include dermatitis, folliculitis, photosensitivity reaction, pruritus, erythema, dry skin, irritation, and *Clostridium difficile*-associated colitis [11]. Adherence to daily application of topical antibiotic agents is as low as 45% [14]. Above-mentioned side effects may lead to poor tolerability of recommended treatment, which has been suggested to reduce patient's adherence. To further investigate this, one study identified 35 studies evaluating tolerability of topical antibiotics in acne treatment. There was no significant correlation between tolerability and discontinuation when assessing the number of discontinuations caused by tolerability across these studies [14]. Common reasons for unintentional nonadherence to topical antibiotics included forgetfulness or lack of knowledge. Patients may also intentionally not adhere to their topical treatment believing their condition may have improved.

Benzoyl Peroxide

Benzoyl peroxide (BP) has bactericidal activity against *C. acnes* through bacterial oxidation, anti-inflammatory properties, and weak activity against comedones [15]. While, current acne treatment guidelines incorporate BP as an important component, acne patients have poor adherence to BP

[11, 16]. Adherence to topical 5% BP ranged from 14–79% when measured using electronic monitoring [17]. A prospective cohort study of 84 patients assessing adherence to physician recommended OTC BP revealed that only 36% of patients included an OTC recommendation when recounting their treatment plan verbally [16].

Salicylic/Azelaic Acids

Salicylic and azelaic acid are OTC acne products, which can be used in combination with other drugs for the symptomatic treatment of mild-to-moderate acne. These treatments may cause side effects that lead to poor adherence, such as excessive erythema, scaling, pruritus, burning, dryness, irritation, and dermatitis [11]. However, a cross-section, Web-based survey of US females ages 25–45 revealed that salicylic acid was the most frequently used (34% of survey respondents) OTC treatment across all racial/ethnic groups [18].

Nonadherence to Systemic Therapy

The treatment of acne often requires more than topical therapy. The systemic medications used in acne management include oral antibiotics, hormonal agents, and oral isotretinoin [11]. Adherence to oral isotretinoin is higher compared to systemic antibiotics and hormonal agents [8, 17, 19].

Patients with acne were more adherent to isotretinoin (71%) than to non-isotretinoin treatments (35%). Another study assessing adherence to isotretinoin estimated adherence rate of approximately 87.5% during the initial course and 60.5% during subsequent courses [10]. Isotretinoin causes many bothersome side effects; while one might predict that side effects would reduce adherence, the presence of bothersome side effects might help prevent patients from forgetting to take the medication. Another possibility is that improved isotretinoin adherence may be attributable to the strict requirements of the iPLEDGE program patients and providers must follow for isotretinoin therapy. The iPLEDGE is a special restricted distribution program approved by the Food and Drug Administration to minimize fetal exposure due to the teratogenic potential of isotretinoin; during treatment, patients are required to have monthly follow-up visits [11].

Interventions to Improve Adherence

Poor adherence to acne treatment is multifactorial and is a main contributor to treatment failure [20]. Barriers to patient adherence include lack of education, poor tolerance of adverse effects, complex treatment plans, low satisfaction, cost of treatment, and busy lifestyle [17, 21, 22]. Interventions to improve patient adherence could target these factors (Table 9.2).

Simplified Regimen

Complex treatment regimens are a barrier to patient adherence [23]. Patients, especially adolescents, are busy. Time-consuming skin care routines are unappealing. Adolescents prefer a simple morning routine, and after-school activities make it difficult to adhere to multiple-dosing regimens [24]. Not only do patients sometimes forget, they may hesitate to use their medication in front of peers. Additionally, patients may not enjoy the feel of layering multiple topical products under their regular

Table 9.2 Studies reporting adherence intervention in acne patients

Study	Sample size	Intervention to increase adherence	Therapy	Length	Measure of adherence	Adherence result
Yentzer et al. [25]	N = 26	Combination therapy once daily versus daily application of 2 separate medications	Combination group: Clindamycin phosphate 7.2% / tretinoin 0.025% gel; control group: Clindamycin phosphate gel 1% and tretinoin cream 0.025%	12 weeks	E-monitoring using MEMS caps	Adherence was 88% in the combination group and 61% in the control group (p = 0.02)
Yentzer et al. [41]	N = 20	Intervention group received internet-based survey as a weekly reminder vs. no reminder in the control group	Daily topical benzoyl peroxide 5% gel	12 weeks	E-monitoring	Median adherence was 74% in the internet group vs. 32% in the control group (p < 0.01)
Yentzer et al. [41]	N = 61	Patients randomized into 4 groups: Standard of care, frequent office visits, daily phone call reminders to patients, daily phone call reminders to patients' parents	Once daily topical therapy	12 weeks	E-monitoring	Median adherence was 82% for frequent office visits, 59% for standard of care, 48% for phone calls to patients, and 36% for phone calls to patients' parents
Boker et al. [39]	N = 40	Intervention group received twice daily text message reminders while the control group did not receive text messages	Clindamycin 1%/benzoyl peroxide 5% gel in the mornings and adapalene 0.3% gel nightly	12 weeks	E-monitoring	Mean adherence was 33.9% in the reminder group and 36.5% in the control group (p = 0.75) with similar clinical improvements in acne severity
Sandoval et al. [32]	N = 17	Intervention group received demonstration on how to use medication vs. control group that received no demonstration	Adapalene/benzoyl peroxide gel once daily	6 weeks	E-monitoring	Median adherence rates were 50% in the sample group compared to 35% in the control group (p = 0.67)
Fabroccini et al. [40]	N = 160	Intervention group received smart phone text messages while control group received no texts.		12 weeks	Self-reported	Adherence improved from 4.10 to 6.6 days per week in the text-message group, and 4.3 to 4.9 in the control group (p < 0.0001)

(continued)

Table 9.2 (continued)

Study	Sample size	Intervention to increase adherence	Therapy	Length	Measure of adherence	Adherence result
Navarette-Dechent et al. [33]	N = 80	Providing a written plan/written counseling in addition to oral counseling in the intervention group vs. oral counseling only in the control group	Combination of topical and systemic therapy	6 months	Self-reported	Adherence was 80% in the intervention group vs. 62% in the control group
Myhill et al. [34]	N = 97	Intervention group received supplementary patient education material (SEM) vs. control group vs. standard-of-care patient education (SOCPE) vs. SOCPE + more frequent office visits	Adapalene 0.1% / benzoyl peroxide 2.5% gel once daily	12 weeks	E-monitoring	Adherence was greatest in the SEM group with a mean of 63.1% (p = 0.0206). Adherence in the SOCPE group and SOCPE plus additional office visits group was 48.2% and 56.5%, respectively

E-monitoring Electronic monitoring, *MEMS* Medication Event Monitoring System

makeup in the morning. Using combination therapies applied nightly prior to bed may offer a solution to this problem [24]. This reduces the number of medications the patient must obtain and store, and decrease the number of steps required for application. The less disruptive the treatment is to the patient's daily routine, the higher the adherence [10].

Simplifying dosing regimens improves treatment outcomes [7, 25, 26]. A randomized study of 26 patients with mild to moderate acne assessed the adherence of combination therapy applied once daily versus daily applications of 2 separate medications for 12 weeks. Patients were randomly assigned to either a combination product group or a control group. The combination group was prescribed clindamycin phosphate 7.2%/tretinoin 0.025% gel to be applied once daily. The control group was assigned clindamycin phosphate gel 1% and tretinoin cream 0.025% to be applied separately, for a total of 2 daily applications. Adherence was monitored with medication event monitoring system caps and severity was assessed at weeks 4, 8, and 12 using acne lesion counts and investigator global assessments. Twenty-one patients completed the study. Adherence was 88% in the combination group and 61% in the control group. After week 12, this difference was statistically significant (P = 0.02) suggesting combination therapy as an effective strategy for improving adherence [25].

Patient Education

Patient education is a key component to adherence [27]. Multiple myths surround the cause of acne. Many tend to place blame on the patient, claiming acne is ultimately the result of patient hygiene and dietary choices. These misunderstandings frequently produce behaviors that worsen the patient's condition and result in increased frustration. A clear explanation of acne etiology and the "why" behind treatment helps dispel misconceptions and improve results [28].

Management of acne requires long-term treatment, but adherence tends to decrease over time and is lowest in the maintenance phase [20, 29]. It is important for patients to understand why maintenance therapy is a crucial component of acne control. Providers can help patients to this realization by proactively educating patients during the initial visit and explaining the importance of each step in the treatment plan [30]. In a multi-center observational study of 428 acne patients in Japan, 73% reported that their physician's explanation of therapy increased their motivation to follow the treatment recommendation [7].

Adolescence is complicated by both the desire for independence and the goal to be accepted by peers. This can work to the provider's advantage when prescribing acne treatment. Advising the patient that the medication will help give them control over their acne provides independence. Informing them that most other teenagers use the same medication fulfills the desire to fit in with their peers [31].

Setting realistic expectations is an important part of patient education. Teenagers want to see immediate results. They are frustrated easily, and may confuse lack of rapid improvement with treatment failure [24]. Additionally, previous failure of over-the-counter supplements promotes a false belief that successful treatment is impossible [7]. Reassurance and proactive patient education increase adolescents' willingness to follow the recommended therapy.

When prescribing treatment, it may be helpful to provide a demonstration for patients on how to correctly apply the medication [32]. To confirm understanding providers may then ask patients to show them how the medication is to be used. To assess the effect of demonstration on adherence, 17 patients were instructed to use adapalene/benzoyl peroxide gel once per day for 6 weeks. Patients were randomized to a sample group that received a demonstration and a control group that received no demonstration. Median adherence was measured using electronic monitoring, efficacy was measured using the Acne Global Assessment (AGA), lesion counts, and the Perceived Medical Condition Self-Management Scale (PMCSMS). Median adherence rates were 50% in the sample group, compared to 35% in the control group (p = 0.67). The median percent improvement in non-inflammatory lesions was 46% in the sample group and 33% for the control group (p = 0.10). Small sample size was a limiting factor of this study. Although the results were not statistically significant, they do suggest that sample demonstrations may have a large effect on adherence behavior [32].

In addition to explaining the treatment, providers may find it helpful to provide their patients with a written plan. In a randomized of study of 80 patients, those who received written counseling in addition to oral counseling showed 80% adherence compared to 62% adherence in the control group (p = 0.043). The written counseling group also received a phone call summarizing instructions within 15 days of initiating treatment. Adherence was assessed through self-reporting after 30, 60, 90 days and 6 months. The study concluded that written counseling improves adherence during the first month of treatment [33].

An additional randomized study of 97 acne patients evaluated the effect of supplementary patient education material (SEM) versus standard-of-care patient education (SOCPE) and SOCPE plus more frequent office visits on treatment adherence and satisfaction. SEM consisted of a short video, information card, and a link to additional information online. SOCPE consisted of oral instructions and a package insert. Patients were prescribed once daily adapalene 0.1%/benzoyl peroxide 2.5% gel then randomized to a SEM group, SOCPE group, or SOCPE plus more frequent office visits group. Adherence was measured using medication electronic monitoring system caps. Additional assessments included a 12-item patient appreciation questionnaire, a 14-week physician questionnaire, and a safety assessment. Adherence was greatest in the SEM group with a mean of 63.1% (p = 0.0206). Adherence in the SOCPE group and SOCPE plus additional office visits group was 48.2% and 56.5%, respectively. Based on the subject appreciation questionnaire, the SEM better helped improve adherence (56.7%) than more visits (32.3%) and SCOPE alone (15.2%). Patients also reported SEM helped them understand how to best use the product (70%) compared to more visits (61.3%) and SCOPE alone (54.5%). The SEM group also reported fewer adverse events. 90% of physicians who participated would consider using SEM in their practice [34].

Reminders

Forgetfulness is a barrier to adherence [19]. Multiple methods can be utilized as reminders for patients. In a meta-analysis of 11 studies, 8 of 11 showed a statistically significant increase in adherence for the reminder group. These trials included phone calls, texts, pagers, video calls, programmed reminder devices and interactive voice response systems [35]. Teenagers' knowledge of technology makes web-based reminders a promising method [36]. Technology-based reminders are feasible and affordable options, although additional research is needed regarding the improvement in adherence surrounding texting and smartphone-based interventions [37].

Evidence suggests texting may be useful for improving adherence, especially when combined with another method [38]. Data is conflicting on whether or not text messages alone are effective in improving adherence. In one randomized study of 40 acne patients prescribed clindamycin/benzoyl peroxide 1%/5% gel in the mornings and nightly adapalene 0.3% gel, 20 patients were assigned to receive twice daily text message reminders. The control group of 20 patients did not receive reminder texts. Fifteen patients in the text group and 18 patients in the control group completed the study. Adherence was measured with electronic Medication Event Monitoring System caps. After 12 weeks the mean adherence was 33.9% in the reminder group and 36.5% in the control group (p = 0.75), with similar clinical improvements in acne severity. Daily text messages did not result in significant differences in adherence to topical medications. Limitations include small sample size, redundant texts, and possible discrepancies between the event monitoring caps and medication application [39]. An additional randomized study evaluated the effect of smart phone short message service (SMS) on acne treatment adherence. One hundred sixty patients participated and were randomly assigned to an SMS group and a control group. The SMS group received 2 texts twice per day and the control group received no texts. At week 0 and after 12 weeks, outcomes were measured using digital photos, the Dermatology Life Quality Index (DLQI), the Global Acne Grading System (GAGS), the Cardiff Acne Disability Index (CADI), Patient-Doctor Depth-of-Relationship Scale, and patient-reported adherence. Patient adherence improved from 4.10 to 6.6 days per week in the SMS group, and 4.3 to 4.9 days per week in the control group. Based on the GAGS score, the patients in the SMS group had better results. Additionally, the DLQI and CADI measurements showed improvement in quality of life for the SMS group. Text messages are an effective strategy to improve patient adherence and satisfaction (p < 0.0001) Limitations include small sample size and patient-reported adherence [40]..

Accountability

A prospective study utilized a 6-question internet-based survey as an accountability intervention. This investigator-blinded, randomized study involved 20 acne patients age 13 to 18 years. Patients were prescribed topical benzoyl peroxide 5% gel to be used daily for 12 weeks. Participants were randomized to a control group and an internet-based survey group. The survey group received a weekly survey via email. Eight patients from the control group and 7 from the survey group complete the study. Median adherence measured via event monitoring caps was 74% in the internet group vs. 32% in the control group (p < 0.01), suggesting an internet survey may be an effective method for improving adherence [41]. The survey may create the sense of accountability that occurs with office visits, thereby increasing adherence [42]. If frequent follow-up appointments are not feasible, surveys may be an appropriate adjunct to improve adherence [5].

Incorporate Treatment with Daily Activity

For treatment to be successful, patients must be willing to use their medication regularly. Complicated, time-consuming treatments disrupt patients' everyday routines while simple regimens are more easily incorporated into activities of daily life. It may be beneficial to ask patients to provide an overview of their daily activities and preference. Some would prefer to apply medications each morning, whereas others find they have the most time before bed. Consideration of these preferences when creating a treatment regimen improves adherence [28].

In addition to simplifying treatments for compatibility, some providers recommend associating acne treatment with a daily activity. Storing the medication near frequently used objects or products can serve as a reminder, especially those that are rarely forgotten. For example, medications could be kept near toothbrush and toothpaste, on nightstands, or with make-up [24].

Vehicles and Devices

Acne medications are available in multiple vehicles including creams, gels, and foams. Since patients may tolerate certain vehicles more than others, giving patients a choice increases adherence [43]. For example, topical retinoids are available in different forms. Tazarotene 0.1% can be prescribed as a gel, cream, or foam. In certain patients who don't tolerate the feel of a gel or cream, the foam vehicle may increase satisfaction and adherence [44].

The delivery system of topical medications may affect ease of use and patient satisfaction. One 15-day, open label study evaluated patient preference for the topical medication delivery system. Three hundred patients were assigned to use adapalene 0.1%/benzoyl peroxide 2.5% gel. The medication was provided in a tube or a pump. After one week, participants switched to the alternative delivery method and used the medication for another 7 days. Preference was measured through a patient survey. Two hundred ninety-one patients completed the survey. 79% preferred the pump and 21% preferred the tube (p = 0.001). 89% thought the pump was easy to use, 73% thought it was clean, and 69% reported the pump as convenient. 92% reported satisfaction with the pump delivery-system and 77% stated they would request the pump the next time the medication was prescribed [45].

Avoid Oppositional Defiant Behaviors

Teens do not want to be told what to do. They want to feel like they have control. It's important to encourage reminders without making adolescents feel defiant. Involving patients in treatment discussions and acknowledging their preferences bolsters independence. Promoting self-management in teens increases adherence and hosts long-term benefits [37].

Due to the oppositional defiant behavior of teens, parent intervention can be counterproductive [38]. Rather than obey a parent's orders to remember their acne treatment, a rebellious teen may refuse the medication in an act of defiance [31]. Giving patients more control over their choice of treatment and reminder system improves adherence [31, 46]. A randomized controlled study of strategies to increase adherence in adolescents found the parental reminder group to have the lowest adherence [41]. This study involved 61 adolescents with moderate to severe acne. Patients were prescribed once daily topical therapy and randomized to one of four groups: standard care, frequent office visits, daily phone call reminders to patients, daily phone call reminders to patients' parents. Adherence was measured via MEMS caps for 12 weeks. Median adherence was 82% for frequent office visits, 59% for standard care, 48% for phone calls to patients, and 36% for phone calls to patients' parents [41].

Frequent Follow-Up

Increasing the frequency of office visits may improve treatment results through "white coat compliance." [42]. Patients tend to change their behavior when they know they are being watched closely, a phenomenon known as Hawthorne effect [47]. This explains why adherence is often higher in clinical trials. Observation of 29 patients enrolled in a clinical trial for psoriasis showed adherence rates improved around the time of office visits (p < 0.05) [42]. Additionally, a randomized study of 61 adolescents with acne investigated the effect of increased frequency of office visits on adherence. Return visits for the standard of care group were scheduled at weeks 6 and 12. Patients in the frequent visit group presented for follow-up weeks 1, 2, 4, 6, 8, and 12. Adherence measured with MEMS caps was 82% in the frequent visit group compared to 59% in the standard of care group [41].

When discussing adherence with patients, indirect questioning, rather than direct questioning, may result in a more accurate assessment of patient adherence. This measure of adherence is often more accurate than relying on long-term memory. "Are you taking your medication?" is a direct question. Indirect questions are less accusatory, for example, "Do you need a refill?" Additional studies are required, but evidence suggests indirect questioning helps prevent patient defensiveness [48].

Improve Patient Satisfaction

Patient satisfaction is a key factor for continued adherence. Patient-physician communication plays a key role in this process [27]. Involving patients in their treatment plans and agreeing on a course of action can positively impact adherence [17]. Interventions personalized to patient or parent needs also improve outcomes. For example, allowing the patient to select the type of vehicle increases the tolerability of the therapy, and therefore increases likelihood they will actually apply the medication [17].

Physicians have a responsibility to address patients' concerns [23]. Poor adherence may be due to frustration over previous treatment failure or fear of side effects [49]. Patients may be more willing to tolerate side effects when they recognize that minor, expected side effects indicate the medication is working as intended. Therefore, educating patients prior to initiating treatment is crucial [49]. The provider can work with the patient to manage uncomfortable adverse effects, such as dryness or irritation with moisturizers and gentle cleansers. Additionally, medications can be formulated to minimize side effects. Clindamycin 1%/benzoyl peroxide 5% is available in combination with a hydrating gel. This combination decreases irritation commonly associated with use of these topical medications [50].

The tolerability and patient satisfaction of a combination of benzoyl peroxide 5% gel with liquid cleanser and an SPF 30 moisturizer was evaluated in an open-label study of 50 participants. Patients >12 years old with mild to moderate acne were prescribed benzoyl peroxide 5% gel once daily, liquid cleanser twice daily, and an SPF moisturizer once daily for 12 weeks. Satisfaction and tolerability were measured using a satisfaction questionnaire, investigator global assessment of improvement, lesion count, presence of *Cutibacterium acnes,* and safety. 87% of patients were satisfied with the regimen. 94% of participants reported increased self-esteem. Reduced irritation and itching relief were reported by 81% and 87%, respectively. The *C. acnes* load was reduced by 89% at week one. The three-part-regimen was well tolerated. 80% of patients believed the cleanser to be a necessary part of treatment along with 84% considering the moisturizer a necessity [21].

Cost is often a barrier to adherence to treatment. This is not always discussed with the physician. To improve primary adherence, providers may warn patients that the medication may be expensive and discuss a back-up plan should the first-line treatment not be available [6].

Physician-patient communication improves patient adherence. According to a cross-sectional survey study of 20,901 evaluated patient satisfaction. This study utilized surveys to measure patient perceptions of empathy portrayed by physicians through their friendliness and caring. Empathy was most predominantly linked to satisfaction with partial correlation of 0.87 (p < 0.001) and a Pearson correlation of 0.92 (p < 0.001). Patients who perceived their physicians as empathetic were more satisfied with their experience, and were therefore more likely to be adherent to the prescribed treatment [51].

Conclusion

Acne medication adherence is poor and a major reason for treatment failure. Nonadherence is particularly prevalent among teenagers who are the majority of acne population. Reasons for poor adherence include complexity of acne treatment, misunderstanding physician's directions, fear of side effects, and forgetfulness. Simplifying treatment regimens, patient education, reminders, frequent follow-up visits are helpful interventions, which may improve treatment adherence and lead to better outcomes and improved quality of life.

Disclosures Feldman has received research, speaking and/or consulting support from a variety of companies including Galderma, GSK/Stiefel, Almirall, Leo Pharma, Boehringer Ingelheim, Mylan, Celgene, Pfizer, Valeant, Abbvie, Samsung, Janssen, Lilly, Menlo, Merck, Novartis, Regeneron, Sanofi, Novan, Qurient, National Biological Corporation, Caremark, Advance Medical, Sun Pharma, Suncare Research, Informa, UpToDate and National Psoriasis Foundation. He is founder and majority owner of www.DrScore.com and founder and part owner of Causa Research, a company dedicated to enhancing patients' adherence to treatment.

Wasim Haidari, Katelyn Glines, and Dr. Cline have no conflicts to disclose.

References

1. Cong TX, Hao D, Wen X, Li XH, He G, Jiang X. From pathogenesis of acne vulgaris to anti-acne agents. Arch Dermatol Res. 2019;311:337–49.
2. Das S, Reynolds RV. Recent advances in acne pathogenesis: implications for therapy. Am J Clin Dermatol. 2014;15(6):479–88.
3. Dreno B, Bordet C, Seite S, Taieb C. Acne relapses: impact on quality of life and productivity. J Eur Acad Dermatol Venereol. 2019;33:937–43.
4. Hosthota A, Bondade S, Basavaraja V. Impact of acne vulgaris on quality of life and self-esteem. Cutis. 2016;98(2):121–4.
5. Moradi Tuchayi S, Alexander TM, Nadkarni A, Feldman SR. Interventions to increase adherence to acne treatment. Patient Prefer Adherence. 2016;10:2091–6.
6. Ryskina KL, Goldberg E, Lott B, Hermann D, Barbieri JS, Lipoff JB. The role of the physician in patient perceptions of barriers to primary adherence with acne medications. JAMA Dermatol. 2018;154(4):456–9.
7. Miyachi Y, Hayashi N, Furukawa F, et al. Acne management in Japan: study of patient adherence. Dermatology (Basel, Switzerland). 2011;223(2):174–81.
8. Tan X, Al-Dabagh A, Davis SA, et al. Medication adherence, healthcare costs and utilization associated with acne drugs in Medicaid enrollees with acne vulgaris. Am J Clin Dermatol. 2013;14(3):243–51.
9. Hester C, Park C, Chung J, Balkrishnan R, Feldman S, Chang J. Medication adherence in children and adolescents with acne vulgaris in Medicaid: a retrospective study analysis. Pediatr Dermatol. 2016;33(1):49–55.
10. Snyder S, Crandell I, Davis SA, Feldman SR. Medical adherence to acne therapy: a systematic review. Am J Clin Dermatol. 2014;15(2):87–94.
11. Zaenglein AL, Pathy AL, Schlosser BJ, et al. Guidelines of care for the management of acne vulgaris. J Am Acad Dermatol. 2016;74(5):945–73.33.
12. Lee IA, Maibach HI. Pharmionics in dermatology: a review of topical medication adherence. Am J Clin Dermatol. 2006;7(4):231–6.
13. Koehler AM, Maibach HI. Electronic monitoring in medication adherence measurement. Implications for dermatology. Am J Clin Dermatol. 2001;2(1):7–12.
14. Bartlett KB, Davis SA, Feldman SR. Topical antimicrobial acne treatment tolerability: a meaningful factor in treatment adherence. J Am Acad Dermatol. 2014;71(3):581–2.. e582
15. Gollnick HP. From new findings in acne pathogenesis to new approaches in treatment. J Eur Acad Dermatol Venereol. 2015;29(Suppl 5):1–7.
16. Huyler AH, Zaenglein AL. Adherence to over-the-counter benzoyl peroxide in patients with acne. J Am Acad Dermatol. 2017;77(4):763–4.
17. Ahn CS, Culp L, Huang WW, Davis SA, Feldman SR. Adherence in dermatology. J Dermatolog Treat. 2017;28(2):94–103.

18. Rendon MI, Rodriguez DA, Kawata AK, et al. Acne treatment patterns, expectations, and satisfaction among adult females of different races/ethnicities. Clin Cosmet Investig Dermatol. 2015;8:231–8.

19. Anderson KL, Dothard EH, Huang KE, Feldman SR. Frequency of primary nonadherence to acne treatment. JAMA Dermatol. 2015;151(6):623–6.

20. Koo J. How do you foster medication adherence for better acne vulgaris management? Skinmed. 2003;2(4):229–33.

21. Kim MR, Kerrouche N. Combination of benzoyl peroxide 5% gel with liquid cleanser and moisturizer SPF 30 in acne treatment results in high levels of subject satisfaction, good adherence and favorable tolerability. J Dermatolog Treat. 2018;29(1):49–54.

22. Gollnick HP, Bettoli V, Lambert J, et al. A consensus-based practical and daily guide for the treatment of acne patients. J Eur Acad Dermatol Venereol. 2016;30(9):1480–90.

23. Devine F, Edwards T, Feldman SR. Barriers to treatment: describing them from a different perspective. Patient Prefer Adherence. 2018;12:129–33.

24. Baldwin HE. Tricks for improving compliance with acne therapy. Dermatol Ther. 2006;19(4):224–36.

25. Yentzer BA, Ade RA, Fountain JM, et al. Simplifying regimens promotes greater adherence and outcomes with topical acne medications: a randomized controlled trial. Cutis. 2010;86(2):103–8.

26. Feneran AN, Kaufman WS, Dabade TS, Feldman SR. Retinoid plus antimicrobial combination treatments for acne. Clin Cosmet Investig Dermatol. 2011;4:79–92.

27. Storm A, Benfeldt E, Andersen SE, Andersen J. Basic drug information given by physicians is deficient, and patients' knowledge low. J Dermatolog Treat. 2009;20(4):190–3.

28. Thiboutot D, Dreno B, Layton A. Acne counseling to improve adherence. Cutis. 2008;81(1):81–6.

29. Carroll CL, Feldman SR, Camacho FT, Manuel JC, Balkrishnan R. Adherence to topical therapy decreases during the course of an 8-week psoriasis clinical trial: commonly used methods of measuring adherence to topical therapy overestimate actual use. J Am Acad Dermatol. 2004;51(2):212–6.

30. Zirwas MJ, Holder JL. Patient education strategies in dermatology: part 1: benefits and challenges. J Clin Aesthet Dermatol. 2009;2(12):24–7.

31. Lewis DJ, Feldman SR. Practical ways to improve patient adherence. San Bernardino: CreateSpace Independent Publishing Platform; 2017.

32. Sandoval LF, Semble A, Gustafson CJ, Huang KE, Levender MM, Feldman SR. Pilot randomized-control trial to assess the effect product sampling has on adherence using adapalene/benzoyl peroxide gel in acne patients. J Drugs Dermatol. 2014;13(2):135–40.

33. Navarrete-Dechent C, Curi-Tuma M, Nicklas C, Cardenas C, Perez-Cotapos ML, Salomone C. Oral and written counseling is a useful instrument to improve short-term adherence to treatment in acne patients: a randomized controlled trial. Dermatol Pract Concept. 2015;5(4):13–6.

34. Myhill T, Coulson W, Nixon P, Royal S, McCormack T, Kerrouche N. Use of supplementary patient education material increases treatment adherence and satisfaction among acne patients receiving adapalene 0.1%/benzoyl peroxide 2.5% gel in primary care clinics: a multicenter, randomized, controlled clinical study. Dermatol Ther. 2017;7(4):515–24.

35. Fenerty SD, West C, Davis SA, Kaplan SG, Feldman SR. The effect of reminder systems on patients' adherence to treatment. Patient Prefer Adherence. 2012;6:127–35.

36. Bass AM, Farhangian ME, Feldman SR. Internet-based adherence interventions for treatment of chronic disorders in adolescents. Adolesc Health Med Ther. 2015;6:91–9.

37. Badawy SM, Kuhns LM. Economic evaluation of text-messaging and smartphone-based interventions to improve medication adherence in adolescents with chronic health conditions: a systematic review. JMIR Mhealth Uhealth. 2016;4(4):e121.

38. Park C, Kim G, Patel I, Chang J, Tan X. Improving adherence to acne treatment: the emerging role of application software. Clin Cosmet Investig Dermatol. 2014;7:65–72.

39. Boker A, Feetham HJ, Armstrong A, Purcell P, Jacobe H. Do automated text messages increase adherence to acne therapy? Results of a randomized, controlled trial. J Am Acad Dermatol. 2012;67(6):1136–42.

40. Fabbrocini G, Izzo R, Donnarumma M, Marasca C, Monfrecola G. Acne smart club: an educational program for patients with acne. Dermatology (Basel, Switzerland). 2014;229(2):136–40.

41. Yentzer BA, Gosnell AL, Clark AR, et al. A randomized controlled pilot study of strategies to increase adherence in teenagers with acne vulgaris. J Am Acad Dermatol. 2011;64(4):793–5.

42. Feldman SR, Camacho FT, Krejci-Manwaring J, Carroll CL, Balkrishnan R. Adherence to topical therapy increases around the time of office visits. J Am Acad Dermatol. 2007;57(1):81–3.

43. Beck LA, Thaci D, Hamilton JD, et al. Dupilumab treatment in adults with moderate-to-severe atopic dermatitis. N Engl J Med. 2014;371(2):130–9.

44. Smith JA, Narahari S, Hill D, Feldman SR. Tazarotene foam, 0.1%, for the treatment of acne. Expert Opin Drug Saf. 2016;15(1):99–103.

45. Rueda MJ. Acne subject preference for pump over tube for dispensing fixed-dose combination adapalene 0.1%-benzoyl peroxide 2.5% gel. Dermatol Ther. 2014;4(1):61–70.
46. Bishay LC, Sawicki GS. Strategies to optimize treatment adherence in adolescent patients with cystic fibrosis. Adolesc Health Med Ther. 2016;7:117–24.
47. Davis SA, Feldman SR. Using Hawthorne effects to improve adherence in clinical practice: lessons from clinical trials. JAMA Dermatol. 2013;149(4):490–1.
48. Alinia H, Feldman SR. Assessing medication adherence using indirect self-report. JAMA Dermatol. 2014;150(8):813–4.
49. Lott R, Taylor SL, O'Neill JL, Krowchuk DP, Feldman SR. Medication adherence among acne patients: a review. J Cosmet Dermatol. 2010;9(2):160–6.
50. Tanghetti E. Fixed-combination clindamycin 1%-benzoyl peroxide 5% hydrating gel: a flexible component of acne management. Cutis. 2009;84(5 Suppl):18–24.
51. Uhas AA, Camacho FT, Feldman SR, Balkrishnan R. The relationship between physician friendliness and caring, and patient satisfaction: findings from an internet-based survey. Patient. 2008;1(2):91–6.
52. Biset N, Lelubre M, Senterre C, et al. Assessment of medication adherence and responsible use of isotretinoin and contraception through Belgian community pharmacies by using pharmacy refill data. Patient Prefer Adherence. 2018;12:153–61.

Chapter 10
Technological Advancements to Promote Adherence

Vignesh Ramachandran, Abigail Cline, and Spencer Hawkins

Introduction

Non-adherence to prescribed medications costs the United States $100–$290 billion USD annually [1]. It also costs lives; an estimated 125,000 deaths and over 10% of hospitalizations are due to non-adherence [2]. Physicians, other healthcare providers, and insurers have vested interests in improving non-adherence. There has been significant research and innovation surrounding the use of various health information technologies to improve adherence [3]. In particular, dermatology has high rates of non-adherence and has a vested interest in exploring technology as a means to improve patient adherence [4, 5].

Technology has become an integral part to how medicine is practiced from the electronic medical record to online communication between providers and patients to even e-prescriptions. In this fashion, technology is ubiquitous in the day-to-day of modern medicine. However, the use of technology as it relates to improving patient adherence is a relatively new concept [6]. Physicians, innovators, and businesspersons alike have delved into this rapidly growing domain of healthcare. These technologies may utilize internet networks, telecommunications, smart phones, physical devices/technologies, and more [7, 8].

In this chapter, we present and discuss some of the technological advancements in medication adherence that can be utilized in dermatology. Such a review may help patients overcome barriers to consistent use of their medications and aid providers in helping their patients improve their health.

V. Ramachandran (✉)
Center for Dermatology Research, Department of Dermatology, Wake Forest School of Medicine, Winston-Salem, NC, USA

A. Cline
Department of Dermatology, Wake Forest School of Medicine, Winston-Salem, NC, USA

S. Hawkins
Department of Dermatology, University of Michigan, Ann Arbor, MI, USA

© Springer Nature Switzerland AG 2020
S. R. Feldman et al. (eds.), *Treatment Adherence in Dermatology*, Updates in Clinical Dermatology, https://doi.org/10.1007/978-3-030-27809-0_10

Methods

A systematic review was conducted using PubMed to curate studies of technology use in promoting adherence or compliance in dermatology. Literature review was performed on February 27, 2019 for studies within the last 10 years (2009–2019) keeping in line with recent literature documenting advancements in this domain. Search terms in PubMed were 'adherence' OR 'compliance' AND 'dermatology'. Titles and abstracts of all papers were read by two independent authors (V.R. and A.C.) for inclusion: (1) full-text manuscripts; (2) interventional clinical studies; (3) studies involving dermatology conditions or skin care (e.g. sunscreen use). Articles were excluded if: (1) interventions did not involve the use of some form of technology; (2) outcomes were not measured to allow for comparison between technology-use and standard of care groups; (3) full-text manuscripts not in English. Disputes were resolved via discussion with a third author (S.R.F).

Overall, 2011 manuscripts were identified by search criteria. After applying inclusion and exclusion criteria to titles and abstracts, 26 manuscripts were deemed appropriate for full-text review. During full-text review of manuscripts, an additional 3 manuscripts were removed based on inclusion/exclusion criteria, resulting in a final count of 23 manuscripts included.

In a non-systematic fashion, newer technologies without many trial data or ancillary studies were searched in a non-systematic fashion using PubMed and Google Scholar. Additionally, Google was used to identify websites discussing various companies' technologies functioning within the realm of patient adherence.

Mobile Phone-Based Technology (mHealth)

Cell phones have become a ubiquitous technology used by two-thirds of the world's population, piquing the interest in healthcare researchers and entrepreneurs in utilizing the technology to improve adherence [9]. The low costs and barriers to engage patients through mobile phone-based technology (mHealth), especially in rural or underserved areas, is particularly intriguing to providers [9]. Text message reminders and phone-based applications are some of the most common reported methods aimed at improving patient adherence. For instance, a meta-analysis of randomized clinical trials of mobile phone text message reminders for patients with chronic diseases managed by internal medicine physicians has shown a near double in odds of medication adherence [10]. Dermatology has also investigated mHealth as a way to improve adherence.

Text Reminders

A randomized controlled study compared adherence in acne patients receiving text message reminders to control in 160 adults over the course of 12 weeks. Eighty patients were randomly assigned to receive two text messages daily (morning and evening) while 80 control patients did not receive any text reminders. Evaluation of patients during the 12-week study period included digital photographs, Global Acne Grading System (GAGS), Dermatology Life Quality Index (DLQI), and Cardiff Acne Disability Index (CADI). Adherence was assessed by seven-day recall questionnaire on the last week of treatment. From beginning to end of the study period, adherence in the text message group increased from 4.10 to 6.6 days/week compared to no significant increase in the control group (4.3–4.9 days/week) (P < 0.0001). GAGS score decreased significantly in the text message group (25.3 ± 8.9 to 8.7 ± 3.6) while there was no significant change in the control group (24.7 ± 7.6 to 16.2 ± 5.6)

(P < 0.0001). DQLI scores in the text message group decreased significantly (9.2 ± 2.2 to 5.4 ± 1.8) compared to no significant change in the control group (9.5 ± 1.8 to 8.0 ± 1.4) (P < 0.0001). CADI scores similarly decreased significantly in the text message group (8.6 ± 1.3 to 2.0 ± 0.8) compared to the control group 7.8 ± 1.2 to 5.0 ± 0.8) (P < 0.0001). Additionally, 65% of patients were "very much satisfied", 30% were "quite satisfied", 4% "not much satisfied" and 1% were "not at all satisfied" with the text message service [11].

A randomized controlled multi-institutional trial compared adherence in acne patients receiving text message reminders to control in 33 healthy patients aged 12–35 years over the course of 12 weeks. Patients were randomized to experimental (n = 15) and control (n = 18) groups. The experimental cohort received customized twice-daily text message reminders to apply acne medication (clindamycin/benzoyl peroxide 1%/5% gel in the mornings and adapalene 0.3% gel in the evenings) while the control group received no such reminder. Electronic monitoring caps were used to assess adherence, the primary outcome measure. The secondary outcome measure was IGSA score and self-reported improvement of acne severity. Mean adherence rate for the text message reminder group was 33.9% compared to control group mean adherence rate of 36.5% (P = 0.75). Despite similar baseline IGSA scores, the text message reminder group had no significantly difference change in scores (2.3 to 1.2) compared to control group (2.4 to 1.6). Furthermore, mean self-reported improvement in acne severity was 55.3% in the text message group compared to 57.5% in the control group. When both groups' data was combined, patients with higher individual adherence demonstrated greater decrease in acne lesion count by end of the 12-week study although this finding was not statistically significant (R^2 = .0613) [12].

A randomized controlled trial compared adherence in children with atopic dermatitis and their caregivers receiving educational and reminder text message reminders to control in 30 children over the course of 42 days. Parents of both groups were provided a quiz at the initial visit and final follow-up visit to assess their knowledge of atopic dermatitis. Eczema Area Severity Index (EASI) scores were also measured at initial visit and follow-up. There was no significant difference in EASI score between the text message (−53% mean decrease) and control (−58% decrease) groups. However, the group receiving text messages scores significantly higher (84% correct) than the control group (75% correct) (P = 0.04) [13]. The authors surmise that the difference in scores were due to patients reading the text message reminders. However, a subjective or objective direct measurement of adherence was not performed but inferred.

A pilot study assessed adherence in atopic dermatitis patients receiving text message reminders and condition-specific educational information texts in 25 children 14 years of age or older over the course of 6 weeks. Outcomes measured included survey of treatment adherence (via 7-day recall and questionnaire assessing how often medication use was forgotten), survey of self-care actions (14 behaviors via Likert scale), disease severity (via SCORing Atopic Dermatitis index, SCORAD), DLQI (17 and older) or Child Dermatology Quality of Life Index (CDQLI, 16 or younger), and usability/satisfaction (0 to 10 scale)with the text message reminder program. All pre-intervention measurements increased post-intervention. Specifically, treatment adherence (mean days/week) increased from 3.8 (SD 2.4) pre-intervention to 6.0 (SD 1.7) post-intervention (P < 0.001). Mean number (days/week) of self-care actions reported as "always" increased from 3.6 (SD 2.3) pre-intervention to 6.1 (SD 3.1) post-intervention (P < 0.002). Mean SCORAD decreased from 33.4 (SD 8.9) pre-intervention to 28.2 (SD 7.7) post-intervention (P < 0.001). Finally, DQLI/CDQLI decreased from 7.8 (SD 5.2) pre-intervention to 5.0 (SD 3.8) post-intervention (P < 0.014). The usefulness/satisfaction of the text message tool was graded as 7.1 (SD 2.4, range 2–10). 88% reported it as useful; 84% wanted to continue in the program; 92% found the educational texts helpful; 84% would recommend such a system to friends; and 72% would pay a small fee for the service [14].

A randomized controlled trial compared adherence in psoriasis patients receiving text message reminders compared to control in 40 patients over the course of 12 weeks. Evaluation of patients during the 12-week study included Psoriasis Area Severity Index (PASI), Self-Administered Psoriasis Area

Severity Index (SAPASI), DLQI, Physician Global Assessment (PGA), patient-physician relationship questionnaire, and treatment adherence. The last outcome was evaluated through a series of multiple-choice questions assessing failure to use medications (days/week) with confirmation via 7-day recall calendar. The text message reminder group showed significantly increased treatment adherence (3.86 days/week to 6.46 days/week) compared to the control group which showed no significant change (P < 0.001). After 12 weeks, the text message reminder group had significant reduction in PASI (P < 0.05), SAPASI (P < 0.05), and PGA (P < 0.05) despite both groups having similar baseline values of each index score. Similarly, DLQI was significantly increased in the text message reminder group compared to the control group (P < 0.05). Likely as a result of the positive disease severity and quality of life scores, patients receiving text message reminders demonstrated improved patient-physician relationship scores compared to the control group, which had similar scores at the beginning and end of the 12-week treatment period (P < 0.01). Overall, 85% found text message reminders useful; 75% would recommend such a service to friends; 75% would continue with the text messages; and 15% would even pay a small fee for such a system to integrate with their psoriasis medications [15].

A randomized controlled trial compared adherence for sunscreen use in patients receiving text message reminders to control in 70 adult patients over the course of 6 weeks. Patients in the text message reminder group received daily reminders entailing a "hook" (regarding daily local weather) and "prompt" (reminder to use sunscreen). The primary outcome measured was adherence to sunscreen by the number of days used over the course of 6 weeks, which was measured by electronic monitoring device. Over the course of the 6 weeks, the text message reminder group maintained similar adherence at the start and end of the study, whereas the control group showed precipitous decline. Specifically, at the end of the 6-week period, the text message reminder group had mean adherence of 23.6 days (95% confidence interval [CI] 20.2–26.9 days) with daily adherence of 56.1% (95% CI: 48.1% to 64.1%) whereas the control group had mean adherence of 12.6 days (95% CI: 9.7–15.5 days) with daily adherence of 30.0% (95% CI: 23.1% to 36.9%). Statistical analysis of both mean adherence days and daily adherence percentages yielded P < 0.001. Although weekly adherence was similar after week one (50% in control group verses 58% in text message reminder group, P = 0.21), thereafter weekly comparisons of adherence were significantly different (P = 0.01 for week 2 and P < 0.001 for weeks 3–6). Sub-analysis of adherence on 8 rainy days (38% text message reminder group versus 9% control group) and 31 cloudy days (55% text message reminder group versus 30% control group) were also significantly increased in the interventional group (both P < 0.001). These results remained after controlling for demographic, educational, age, and other patient characteristics. A mean score of 8.31 (standard deviation [SD] of 1.99) out of 10 was reported for the utility of the reminder system (0 = not useful at all; 10 = most useful). 69% of participants would continue with reminders while 89% would recommend it to friends [16].

Another randomized controlled trial compared adherence to sunscreen use in three groups of patients (including one group receiving text message reminders) in 149 adults over the course of 12 weeks. All three groups received sun protection advice. Group 1 received 4000 HUF in compensation at the conclusion of 12 weeks. Group 2 received free sun protection factor (SPF) 50+ sunscreen. Group 3 (experimental) group received the SPF 50+ sunscreen and were sent personalized educational e-mails and text messages weekly. Adherence was measured by sun exposure diaries and interview results. Group 3 members used sunscreen more often (3.21 days/week ±2.37) than participants of Group 1 (1.47 ± 1.91) and Group 2 (2.09 ± 1.85) (P < 0.005 for both) [17].

Overall, it appears that the frequency of text messaging is not as important as the use of a reminder system itself. For instance, one of the prior mentioned studies showed twice daily text messages did not improve adherence [12]. Meanwhile, another study demonstrated merely weekly text message reminders were sufficient to improve adherence [17]. Too many notifications can lead to alarm fatigue. What may be most important is the context of the messages. A "hook" that provides value to the patient in a manner relative to behavior (e.g. weather or ultraviolet index) in addition to the reminder may be most effective [16].

Telecommunications/Mobile Phone Calls

A seemingly simple modality, phone calling is as accessible of a measure studied to improve adherence in our age of mobile phones.

An open-label, randomized study compared clinical improvement in 12 patients with atopic dermatitis who had previously failed topical corticosteroids under conditions designed to promote good adherence over the course of 7 days. Patients were given desoximethasone spray 0.25% as treatment. They were then randomized to control (n = 6) and experimental group (n = 6), which received twice-daily phone calls to discuss treatment adherence. Outcomes measured were the Pruritus Visual Analog Scale (PVAS), Total Lesion Severity Scale (TLSS), EASI, and Investigator Global Assessment (IGA). Overall, 100% (12/12) showed improvement in PVAS; 83.3% (10/12) showed improvement in EASI score; 75.0% (9/12) showed improvement in TLSS score; and 58.3% (7/12) showed improvement in IGA score. The interventional group receiving twice-daily phone calls showed greater improvement in all parameters compared to control group except for pruritus: PVAS (76.9% in interventional versus 87.0% in control); EASI (46.9% in interventional versus 21.1% in control); TLSS (38.3% in interventional versus 9.7% in control); IGA (45.8% versus 4.2% in control). These dramatic differences were attributed to increased adherence to treatment regimen as a result of phone call reminders [18].

A randomized controlled trial compared adherence in psoriasis patients receiving motivational phone calls compared to control in 177 adults over the course of 6 months. The motivational phone calls were administered at three points during the study (weeks 2, 8, and 16). Outcomes measured were PASI, adherence, and proper application of medication. Baseline characteristics between the two groups were similar. Improvement in PASI was seen in both motivational phone call group (6.8 to 4.8, $P < 0.001$) and control group (7.0 to 5.5, $P < 0.001$). However, there was no statistically difference in reduction between the groups upon completion of the study ($P = 0.136$). No statistically significant difference was seen between the groups to either topical ($P = 0.278$), scalp ($P = 0.250$), or systemic therapy adherence ($P = 0.975$). However, sub-analysis demonstrated patients' proper administration/application of treatment was significantly improved in the motivation phone call group (82.4%) compared to the control group (67.4%) ($P = 0.021$) [19].

An open-label randomized controlled trial comparing adherence in acne patients undergoing different modalities of reminders to control in 46 teenagers was conducted over the course of 12 weeks. All 46 patients were treated with once-daily adapalene gel 0.1%. Four interventional groups were created: Group 1 (standard of care); Group 2 (frequent office visits: weeks 1, 2, 4, 6, 8, and 12); Group 3 (patients received daily phone call reminders); and Group 4 (parents received daily phone call reminders). Adherence was monitored by electronic monitoring caps. Adherence decreased over the study period for all groups. However, the overall difference in adherence was different between the four groups ($P < 0.05$). Group 2 has the highest median adherence (82), followed by Group 1 (59%), Group 3 (48%), and Group 4 (36%) [20].

Smartphone Applications

A randomized controlled trial compared adherence in 134 psoriasis patients using a smartphone application to control was conducted over the course of 28 days. The results of this trial are pending publication. Highlighted are principles of the investigation. In this trial, all patients were treated with topical calcipotriol and betamethasone dipropionate. The application under investigation is a combination of an electronic monitoring unit linked to a smartphone application. The three functions it is meant to serve are: a) provide patients with data on medication consumption; b) measure severity of psoriasis by completing a symptom and photo diary via the application; and c) support patients via reminders to refill medications and optional educational and motivational text messages. Primary outcome measures were rates of adherence measured by patient self-reporting, weight of medication, and electronic monitoring unit data. Secondary outcomes were DQLI and Lattice System Physician's Global Assessment (LS-PGA) scores [21].

Investigation in other fields have showed mixed results. For instance, a randomized controlled trial compared adherence to antidepressant medications in 40 college students who were reminded via a smartphone reminder app (n = 20) or control (n = 20) over the course of 8 weeks. The primary outcome measure was adherence to the medication as measured by dividing the actual number of pills taken by the expected number of pills taken during the study period and multiplying the total by 100. Secondary outcomes included depression scores as measured by Beck Depression Inventory (BDI). Results showed the reminder app group patients were nearly 3.5 times more likely to adhere to their regimen than control group patients; however, these results were not statistically significant (P = 0.057). Similarly, the reduction in BDI scores were not significantly different between interventional (5.50 ± 8.34) and control (3.30 ± 5.40) groups (P = -0.374) [22].

Weekly treatments may be more difficult for patients than daily medications. Smartphones are capable of setting reminders based on standard features already available without additional application downloads. For instance, alarm reminders may be set at a specified time or a reminder notification may be delivered through text form via the reminder icon built-in application on smartphones [23].

It appears reminder apps seems to lose efficacy over time when reminders become ignored. In order to optimize long-term use, such apps may need to use a "hook" to capture patients' attention with a follow-up "reminder" or link reminders to daily behaviors. Additionally, in-productive and recently released are applications created by pharmaceutical companies to serve as reminder systems. It may be prudent for clinicians and researchers to formally assess their utility and design moving forward.

Electronic Health (eHealth)

While eHealth caries similarities to mHealth and overlap may exist (especially with the use of mobile phone technologies to access Internet-based programs), eHealth is much more concerned with the use of computers and networks in healthcare. Use of such components of technology have been used in dermatology to promote adherence.

Web-Based Patient Education

A randomized controlled study comparing knowledge of condition and self-reported adherence in psoriasis patients receiving a web-based psoriasis education application to control in 22 patients was conducted during single office visits. A new training module was developed on DermPatientEd.com, a dermatology patient education webpage, to have an educational video regarding psoriasis, text-based content, and graphics on side effects. During the first clinic visit, patients were randomized to receive a link to the webpage followed by administration of an online quiz or solely access to the online quiz. Outcomes measured were quiz score and self-reported adherence. The web-based education group had a mean score of 11/14 on the psoriasis knowledge quiz compared to the control group mean score of 9/14 (P = 0.007). However, no improvements in self-reported medication adherence were observed [24].

A randomized controlled study compared adherence to sunscreen protection in 93 adult patients receiving online video education to control over the course of 12 weeks. Outcomes measured were assessment of sun protective behavior (using the National Health and Nutrition Examination Survey, NHANES), assessment of sunscreen knowledge (using questionnaire), and satisfaction survey (10-point scale). The experimental cohort received access to the online video, which discussed the mechanism of sunscreens, types of sunscreens, their importance, and proper application. The control group received the same information but as a pamphlet. Over the 12-week study, the online video group showed significant increase in adherence (days/week) to sunscreen use (1.7 ± 2.5 to 3.4 ± 2.6) ($P < 0.005$), unlike the pamphlet group (2.0 ± 3.0 to 2.4 ± 3.0) ($P = 0.552$). There was also a significant difference in the knowledge score increases between the online video group (2.0 ± 1.5) compared to the pamphlet group (1.2 ± 1.0) ($P = 0.003$). Finally, the online video group was significantly more satisfied with their education material (9 ± 0.9) compared to the pamphlet group (7.9 ± 1.3) ($P < 0.001$) [25].

A randomized controlled trial compared the utility of appearance-based video or a health-based video promoting sunscreen use in 50 high school students aged 13 and older. The appearance-based video focused on the negative effects of ultraviolet radiation (e.g. photoaging, wrinkles, sagging skin, uneven tone) whereas the health-based video focused on skin cancer risk and similar concepts. The production quality of both the appearance-based video (7.8 ± 1.3) and the health-based video (8.1 ± 1.3) were similar ($P = 0.676$). The satisfaction survey was administered 6 weeks after viewing the video. Mean satisfaction score for the appearance-based video (8.1 ± 1.2) was significantly higher than the health-based video (6.4 ± 1.4) ($P < 0.001$). Additionally, the mean appeal score for the appearance-based video (8.3 ± 1.0) was significantly higher than the health-based vide (6.6 ± 1.6) ($P < 0.001$) [26]. These authors also conducted a randomized controlled trial in the same patient population compared adherence to sunscreen based on appearance-based or health-based video education. While the health-based group showed a non-statistically significant increase (measured as days/week) in sunscreen use (0.9 ± 1.9, $P = 0.096$), the appearance-based group had a statistically significant increase (2.8 ± 2.2, $P < 0.001$). Inter-group comparison showed that the appearance-based group has significantly higher frequency of sunscreen use compared to the health-based group (2.2 ± 1.4 vs 0.2 ± 0.6, $P < 0.001$) [27].

A randomized controlled trial compared symptom improvement, quality of life, and adherence in 95 high school acne patients receiving automated online counseling to control standard website over the course of 12 weeks. The automated online counseling was an online module system that provides pre-recorded answers to an abundant number of specific questions patients may have. Outcomes measured were assessments of acne severity, quality of life (CDLQI), and skin care behavior. The automated online counseling webpage had the same information as that found in the standard website. There was not a significant difference in the reduction of acne lesions (mean) between the standard website group (21.33 ± 10.81 to 21.13 ± 14.42) and the automated-counseling website group (25.33 ± 12.45 to 21.43 ± 10.69) (between groups $P = 0.10$). Similarly, there was not a significant difference in the reduction in CDLQI scores between the standard website group (2.72 ± 3.19 to 2.54 ± 2.78) and the automated-counseling website group (2.69 ± 3.28 to 2.31 ± 2.99) (between groups $P = 0.71$). However, there was a significant difference in the percentage of patients in the automated-counseling website group (43%, 21/49) who maintained or recently adopted an anti-acne skin care program compared to the standard website group (22%, 10/46) ($P = 0.03$) [28].

Internet-Based Surveys

A randomized controlled trial compared treatment outcomes in 15 acne patients receiving Internet-based surveys compared to control over the course of 12 weeks. All patients were treated with daily topical benzoyl peroxide, 5% gel. The survey group received weekly surveys via e-mail with questions gauging adherence, ease of treatment regimen, efficacy, and side effects experienced. Adherence was also monitored objectively with electronic monitoring caps. Acne Global Assessment scores were used to score improvement at baseline, week 6, and week 12. Overall, the median adherence in the survey group was 74% compared to 32% in the control group (P = 0.01). Additionally, mean adherence dropped quickly (P = 0.02) while the survey group had no significant change in adherence over the study period (P = 0.10). The survey group also demonstrated greater decrease in acne severity as measured by non-inflammatory (44% versus 11%) and total lesion (36% versus 13%) counts, although these results were not statistically significant [29].

This concept has been translated into clinical practice by Causa Research, a company focused on targeting adherence issues facing physicians. Causa Research offers online survey platforms to improve patient adherence [30].

Teledermatology

A randomized controlled study comparing efficacy and adherence to actinic keratosis treatment in 157 patients undertaking care via teledermatology to face-to-face (i.e. in-person) visits was conducted over 4 weeks. Teledermatology visits began with the very first encounter for patients in the interventional group and then repeated at 4 weeks. All patients were prescribed 5% imiquimod applied three times per week. Eight weeks after beginning treatment, a blinded dermatologist assessed clinical response noted as partial, complete, or no response. Outcome measures were percentage of global response (complete response plus partial response) and reasons for treatment failure. Analysis was conducted under per-protocol and intention-to-treat parameters. Under per-protocol analysis, complete response was observed in 65.6% of teledermatology patients compared to 66.7% of face-to-face patients (P > 0.05). Under intention-to-treat analysis, complete response was seen in 51.2% of teledermatology patients and 64.0% of face-to-face patients (P = 0.073), Global response was improved in the face-to-face group (84.0%) compared to the teledermatology group (70.7%) (P = 0.036). However, multivariate analysis showed that the modality of care (face-to-face visits versus teledermatology) was not associated with global response but facial lesions and adverse events did. To assess adherence, reasons for failed therapy were assessed. Face-to-face patients completed the therapy 90.7% of the time compared to 72.0% in teledermatology patients. The major driven of treatment failure in teledermatology patients was not starting the therapy (47.8%) [31]. It is also worth noting, the 4-week study period is not the usual time span of treatment for actinic keratoses in daily practice. Typically, follow-up visits would occur much later.

However, it is plausible that a hybrid approach may exist in the future in which the initial visit is face-to-face (which may also avoid issues such as treatment initiation as noted in the prior mentioned study) with early follow-up via teledermatology to assess response and adherence.

Physical Technologies/Devices

Technology may come in the form of devices which may increase adherence. Typically, these devices serve as a mechanical means to assist, remind, or make it easier for patients to administer their treatments.

A randomized controlled study compared sunscreen adherence in an interventional group given combined sunscreen and toothpaste storage unit to control group (sunscreen only) in 62 Caucasian adult women over the course of 6 weeks. At the initial visit, all patients were advised of the benefits of sunscreen. Thereafter, patients were randomized into Group A (sunscreen only) or Group B (sunscreen + toothpaste storage unit). The outcome measure was difference in weight of sunscreen given at the initial visit (pre- minus post-study weight). The mean pre-weight of sunscreens was 112.2 g for all 62 patients. Group A sunscreen usage was 37.0 g (SD 17.2) while it was 44.1 g (SD 18.0) (P = 0.06). While the difference was not significantly different, it does represent a nearly 20% difference in use over the brief 6-week study [32].

A prospective study compared application success of compression stocking donning in 40 patients over 65 years old with chronic venous insufficiency randomized to order of compression stocking and donning device pairings. Compression stockings studied were one 40 mmHg or two superimposed 20 mmHg models. Donning devices were also studied. The endpoint of the study was successful donning of the compression stocking. Without donning devices, success rate for the one 40 mmHg stockings was 60% (24/40) and 70% (28/40) for patients donning the two superimposed 20 mmHg stockings (P = 0.220). With donning devices, the success rate for 40 mmHg stockings increased to between 88% (35/40; P = 0.001) to 90% (36/40; P = 0.002) depending on the donning device. Similarly, success rate increased to 88% (35/40; P = 0.016) for the two superimposed 20 mmHg stockings. These results were maintained even after controlling for patient characteristics associated with increased success (grip strength, P < 0.05; ability to access forefoot with hand, P = 0.001) [33]. The authors posit adherence is related to ability to don the garment and such devices would increase adherence.

A randomized, double-blinded, placebo-controlled, parallel-group trial compared adherence to secukinumab biologic treatment based on different administration modalities in 220 patients with moderate-to-severe psoriasis over the course of 48 weeks. Patients were assigned to secukinumab 300 mg, secukinumab 150 mg, or placebo at baseline (patients achieving PASI 75 at week 12 were continued on placebo or otherwise started on one of the other two regimens). All patients self-administered the medication or placebo via autoinjector. While the primary outcome of interest to the investigators was clinical efficacy (as measured by PASI and IGA), a secondary measure pertinent to this chapter was patient satisfaction and usability of the autoinjector device (measured by Self-Injection Assessment Questionnaire, SIAQ). This survey assessed feelings about self-injection, self-confidence, and satisfaction with self-injection. After completion of the 48-week study, SIAQ scores for the entire cohort were 8.92, 9.02 and 9.23 for feeling about injections, self-confidence and satisfaction with self-injection, respectively. These represented increases of 1.11 for feeling about injection, 1.70 for self-confidence and 2.52 for satisfaction with self-injection from baseline. 99.4% of patients reported that they were comfortable self-injecting at home (without staff supervision) using the auto-injector device even after the first administration [34].

Another apparent technology present in everyday life are smartwatches, which are increasingly being investigated for utility as medical care adjuncts. These devices are able to provide timely notifications to individuals. However, they lack formal scientific investigation to assess their impact on adherence behaviors.

Multimodal Approaches

A randomized controlled trial compared adherence in 1790 adult psoriasis patients undergoing a multimodal adherence program to control (standard of care) over the course of 64 weeks. All patients were treated with calcipotriol/betamethasone gel. The multimodal adherence program, named Topical Treatment Optimization Programme (TTOP), was comprised of five-elements: guidance for the conversation between dermatologists and patients, guidance for the conversation between nurses and patients, patient information material, telephone/e-mail helpdesks and treatment reminders. Outcomes measured were response to treatment (PGA score of 0 or 1 after 8 weeks of treatment) and patient-reported outcomes (DLQI and Topical Therapy Adherence Questionnaire [TTAQ]). From baseline to week 8, patients in the TTOP arm showed no significant difference in number of days of treatment use compared to the non-TTOP arm (53.5 ± 9.9 versus 53.5 ± 10.2 days). Patients in the non-TTOP group has higher mean use of study medication (adjusted for body surface area) compared to TTOP patients. Both groups showed large variations in usage highlighted by large SD. After 8 weeks, the percentage of patients attaining target response (PGA 0 or 1) was significantly higher for the TTOP group (36.3%) than the non-TTOP group (31.3%, P = 0.0267). After 8 weeks, the mean decrease in DLQI was similar between the TTOP group (2.6 ± 3.7) and non-TTOP group (2.2 ± 3.4). TTAQ responses were significantly higher in TTOP group patients who reported higher rates of feeling well-informed about their disease, treatment, and adherence-related factors (all P < 0.05). Despite the technologic aspects of the program (e.g. automated text message reminders), patients found structured one-to-one conversations with their providers as the most important in TTOP [35].

A multicenter, prospective, open-label interventional study compared efficacy and treatment adherence of a novel ultraviolet B home phototherapy system to control in six patients with stable plaque psoriasis over the course of 10 weeks. The primary outcome measures were Psoriasis Severity Index (PSI) and adherence. The compact technology allowed for home phototherapy and was synchronized to a smartphone application providing treatment plan information (schedule and dosing) and adherence data to the provider. Control lesions (n = 9) had mean change in PSI of 0.67 (95% CI: −0.27 to 1.61) compared to study lesions (n = 9), which had mean change in PSI of 4.44 (95% CI: 2.95 to 5.94) (P < 0.0002). Patient adherence was 96% and treatment satisfaction was 5/5 as rated by 100% of participants [36].

Emerging Concepts

Many of the previously discussed applications of technology to promote adherence pivot existing technological concepts towards tackling adherence issues in medicine and dermatology specifically. In this next section, we will highlight some of the emerging concepts in adherence research and technology that provide new avenues to apply these countermeasures. While many of these technologies are interesting takes on this age-old dilemma, it is important to bear in mind integration of such modalities is of utmost important. Otherwise, alarm fatigue, asynchrony between systems, and complexity of managing the technologies may lead to worse adherence.

Furthermore, integration of these technologies and concepts into the electronic medical record may proove to be a boom for healthcare providers and their patients. By doing so, physicians can assess real-time adherence data and make calculated adjustments or changes to medication regimens. Furthermore, it may downstream aid insurance companies in stratifying risk and insurance premiums/costs for patients. And, most importantly, for patients it would allow for their physician to provide them with personalized and thorough management recommendations.

Gamification

Gamification refers to the concept of applying game playing features (e.g. points, competition) to other realms to promote engagement. This concept has been studied as a psychosocial principle that may be incorporated into technology to promote patient adherence. Literature on this topic is limited. Our literature review revealed 37 papers in PubMed; however, 7 were review papers (18.9%) and 26 (70.3%) were theoretical frameworks/description of app designs without intervention. Herein, we highlight one of the remaining studies, a randomized control study, within the scope of this chapter.

A randomized controlled trial compared intrinsic motivation and physical activity adherence in 36 patients with type 2 diabetes mellitus to control over the course of 24 weeks. Thirty-six inactive, overweight type 2 diabetes patients (45–70 years of age) were randomly assigned to the intentional group, which were instructed to play the smartphone app created by an interdisciplinary team, or control group. Primary outcome was intrinsic physical activity motivation measured by the Intrinsic Motivation Inventory (IMI). From baseline, intrinsic physical activity motivation (IMI score) increased significantly in the study group (+6.4, SD 4.2, $P < 0.001$) compared to the control group in which IMI score decreased (-1.9, SD 16.5, $P = 0.625$) (difference between groups, $P = 0.029$). This increase in IMI score in the interventional group was associated with increased usage of the app ($P = 0.01$; $R^2 = 0.34$). Additionally, IMI score was associated with physical activity level, which was significantly higher in the interventional group compared to control group ($P < 0.05$) [37].

Gamification is an interesting principle that may be applied to adherence. It is a relatively novel concept, but has been highly utilized in the smartphone app space. A systematic review analyzing health and fitness apps related to physical activity and diet in the Apple App Store revealed 132 apps using concepts of gamification. Overall, 121/132 of the apps (91.7%) lacked citations or links to reputable sources to verify the health benefits and information claimed. Further evidence-based literature is needed to assess the utility of gamification [38]. Utilizing patients are resources in creation of these apps may be beneficial.

Automated Medication Dispensers

Traditionally, patients have utilized pill boxes or similar storage devices to medications to aid in daily adherence. While these serve as a memory device, they have shortcomings, such as lack of automation to facilitate memory.

A long-term, prospective feasibility study compared adherence in 21 elderly patients with chronic medical conditions with an automated medication dispenser to baseline adherence over the course of 6 months. All patients were referred by their primary care physician due to poor adherence and for inclusion in the study. Pill counts at baseline determined previous adherence, which was 49.0% for the cohort. Medication adherence was then assessed using an automated home medication dispenser. The dispenser is a bulk-loaded, single-patient medication tool designed to dispense scheduled and as-needed medications in residence. Audio and visual reminders are integrated into the device. Upon completion of the six-month study, adherence was measured at 96.8%, which was significantly higher than baseline ($P < 0.001$) [39].

The results of the prior study have inspired entrepreneurial ventures using this model. For instance, Pillo, Inc. is a company that has engineered a novel automated pill dispenser that combines concepts from machine learning, face recognition, video conferencing, and automation to serve as an overall in-home health assistant that also happens to dispense vitamins and medications [40]. Similarly, MySafeRx™ is a mobile technology integrating concepts such as motivational coaching, adherence monitoring, and electronic pill dispensing to manage office-based opioid treatment using buprenorphine/naloxone. It has demonstrated efficacy early on in a clinical trial before the adherence benefit was lost after conclusion of the study [41].

Some of these companies have technology integrating into medication packs monitoring adherence and provides alerts when doses are missed. Additionally, trusted family members may be notified to encourage adherence. These features may serve as cutting-edge countermeasures, although further research is needed.

Blister Pack Daily Medications

An innovative spin on the age-old distribution of medications, personalized daily medication blister packs are produced by some pharmacies to assist adherence. In this system, the patient's pharmacy places daily medications into small packages labelled with the time and date for when the medications are to be taken. In doing so, it relieves patients of hassles such as personally obtaining medications (which are shipped), identifying them, sorting them, and remembering when in the day to take them (times are labelled on the package). However, this concept does have it shortcomings. It does not necessarily remove the rate-limiting step of patients (and particularly the elderly) remembering to take their medications.

Artificial Intelligence

Artificial intelligence (AI) is one of the hottest technology concepts in our modern world and its permeation into medicine has been inevitable. AI has the potential to assist physicians with diagnostics, procedures, and more. However, it also has a role in adherence.

Google LLC, for instance, has an artificial intelligence/natural language automated calling tool that is live in most of the United States. It is currently used to automate calls to book appointments and similar functions so that the user does not need to. It is not unreasonable to imagine such AI technologies could be educated to provide management recommendations for chronic diseases, call patients to confirm adherence to medications, and follow-up on questions patients may have about their regimens.

Conclusion

Adherence is among the most complicated issues physicians tackle in medicine. Technology has become a focal point in the battle against non-adherence. Many of these technologies utilize existing technologies that patients are generally familiar with (e.g. internet, smartphone apps, pre-existing smartphone reminder capabilities), allowing for ease in integrating these technologies. Other advancements may use new devices/technologies (e.g. at-home phototherapy) or pre-existing technology in a new context (e.g. gamification).

The evolving breadth of advancements in technologies promoting adherence is exciting for medicine and dermatology. However, it is important to realize, fundamentally, adherence is complex and concepts regarding behavior, psychosocial factors, and understanding are crucial regardless of intervention. This may, in part, explain why some of the newer technologies utilize behavior change/behavioral economics and psychological frameworks (e.g. gamification). Additionally, some of the largest barriers to adherence involve access to medication. Indeed, prohibitive costs, difficulties in navigating insurance, and inability to fill prescriptions at pharmacies are some of the largest barriers. Some initiatives have aimed to target such fundamental "gate-keeper" barriers that prelude medication adherence concerns in patients who have their medications [42]. Technological advancements seem to promote adherence despite some mixed results, but it is unquestionable that for any technology to function as expected a strong physician-patient relationship is needed as well as a thorough understanding of the factors contributing to individual non-adherence. Furthermore, patient preferences and characteristics that may limit participation in technologies (e.g. elderly) should be considered.

In other for these technologies to reach their full potential, integration between them and into the electronic medical record may be vital.

Funding sources None

Conflicts of Interest Mr. Vignesh Ramachandran, Dr. Abigail Cline, and Dr. Hawkins have no conflicts of interest to disclose.

References

1. Rosenbaum L, Shrank WH. Taking our medicine — improving adherence in the accountability era. N Engl J Med. 2013;369(8):694–5. https://doi.org/10.1056/NEJMp1307084.
2. McCarthy R. The price you pay for the drug not taken. Bus Health. 1998;16(10):27–8, 30, 32-33. http://www.ncbi.nlm.nih.gov/pubmed/10185113. Accessed February 16, 2019.
3. Nieuwlaat R, Wilczynski N, Navarro T, et al. Interventions for enhancing medication adherence. Cochrane Database Syst Rev. 2014;(11) https://doi.org/10.1002/14651858.CD000011.pub4.
4. Furue M, Onozuka D, Takeuchi S, et al. Poor adherence to oral and topical medication in 3096 dermatological patients as assessed by the Morisky Medication Adherence Scale-8. Br J Dermatol. 2015;172(1):272–5. https://doi.org/10.1111/bjd.13377.
5. Ali SM, Brodell RT, Balkrishnan R, Feldman SR. Poor adherence to treatments. Arch Dermatol. 2007;143(7):912–5. https://doi.org/10.1001/archderm.143.7.912.
6. Mistry N, Keepanasseril A, Wilczynski NL, Nieuwlaat R, Ravall M, Haynes RB. Technology-mediated interventions for enhancing medication adherence. J Am Med Inform Assoc. 2015;22(e1):e177–93. https://doi.org/10.1093/jamia/ocu047.
7. Svendsen MT, Andersen F, Andersen KE. eHealth Technologies as an intervention to improve adherence to topical antipsoriatics: a systematic review. J Dermatolog Treat. 2018;29(2):123–8. https://doi.org/10.1080/09546634.2017.1341612.
8. Hamine S, Gerth-Guyette E, Faulx D, Green BB, Ginsburg AS. Impact of mHealth chronic disease management on treatment adherence and patient outcomes: a systematic review. J Med Internet Res. 2015;17(2):e52. https://doi.org/10.2196/jmir.3951.
9. Akter S, Ray P. mHealth – an ultimate platform to serve the unserved. Yearb Med Inform. 2018;19:94–100. https://doi.org/10.1055/s-0038-1638697.
10. Thakkar J, Kurup R, Laba TL, et al. Mobile telephone text messaging for medication adherence in chronic disease a meta-analysis. JAMA Intern Med. 2016;176:340. https://doi.org/10.1001/jamainternmed.2015.7667.
11. Fabbrocini G, Izzo R, Donnarumma M, Marasca C, Monfrecola G. Acne smart club: an educational program for patients with acne. Dermatology. 2014;229(2):136–40. https://doi.org/10.1159/000362809.
12. Boker A, Feetham HJ, Armstrong A, Purcell P, Jacobe H. Do automated text messages increase adherence to acne therapy? Results of a randomized, controlled trial. J Am Acad Dermatol. 2012;67:1136–42. https://doi.org/10.1016/j.jaad.2012.02.031.
13. Singer HM, Levin LE, Morel KD, Garzon MC, Stockwell MS, Lauren CT. Texting atopic dermatitis patients to optimize learning and eczema area and severity index scores: a pilot randomized control trial. Pediatr Dermatol. 2018;35(4):453–7. https://doi.org/10.1111/pde.13510.
14. Pena-Robichaux V, Kvedar JC, Watson AJ. Text messages as a reminder aid and educational tool in adults and adolescents with atopic dermatitis: a pilot study. Dermatol Res Pract. 2010;2010:1–6. https://doi.org/10.1155/2010/894258.
15. Balato N, Megna M, Di Costanzo L, Balato A, Ayala F. Educational and motivational support service: a pilot study for mobile-phone-based interventions in patients with psoriasis. Br J Dermatol. 2013;168(1):201–5. https://doi.org/10.1111/j.1365-2133.2012.11205.x.
16. Armstrong AW, Watson AJ, Makredes M, Frangos JE, Kimball AB, Kvedar JC. Text-message reminders to improve sunscreen use: a randomized, controlled trial using electronic monitoring. Arch Dermatol. 2009;145:1230–6. https://doi.org/10.1001/archdermatol.2009.269.
17. Szabó C, Ócsai H, Csabai M, Kemény L. A randomised trial to demonstrate the effectiveness of electronic messages on sun protection behaviours. J Photochem Photobiol B Biol. 2015;149:257–64. https://doi.org/10.1016/j.jphotobiol.2015.06.006.
18. Okwundu N, Cardwell LA, Cline A, Unrue EL, Richardson IM, Feldman SR. Topical corticosteroids for treatment-resistant atopic dermatitis. Cutis. 2018;102(3):205–9. http://www.ncbi.nlm.nih.gov/pubmed/30372711. Accessed March 28, 2019.

19. Alpalhão M, Antunes J, Gouveia A, et al. A randomized controlled clinical trial to assess the impact of motivational phone calls on therapeutic adherence in patients suffering from psoriasis. Dermatol Ther. 2018;31(5):e12667. https://doi.org/10.1111/dth.12667.

20. Yentzer BA, Gosnell AL, Clark AR, et al. A randomized controlled pilot study of strategies to increase adherence in teenagers with acne vulgaris. J Am Acad Dermatol. 2011;64(4):793–5. https://doi.org/10.1016/j.jaad.2010.05.008.

21. Svendsen MT, Andersen F, Andersen KH, Andersen KE. Can an app supporting psoriasis patients improve adherence to topical treatment? A single-blind randomized controlled trial. BMC Dermatol. 2018;18(1):2. https://doi.org/10.1186/s12895-018-0071-3.

22. Hammonds T, Rickert K, Goldstein C, et al. Adherence to antidepressant medications: a randomized controlled trial of medication reminding in college students. J Am Coll Heal. 2015;63(3):204–8. https://doi.org/10.1080/07448481.2014.975716.

23. Lin K, Lipner SR. Mobile phone reminders for onychomycosis medication adherence. J Am Acad Dermatol. 2018;80:e105–7. https://doi.org/10.1016/j.jaad.2018.11.010.

24. Hawkins SD, Barilla S, Feldman SR. Web app based patient education in psoriasis – a randomized controlled trial. Dermatol Online J. 2017;23(4). http://www.ncbi.nlm.nih.gov/pubmed/28541882. Accessed March 29, 2019.

25. Armstrong AW, Idriss NZ, Kim RH. Effects of video-based, online education on behavioral and knowledge outcomes in sunscreen use: a randomized controlled trial. Patient Educ Couns. 2011;83(2):273–7. https://doi.org/10.1016/j.pec.2010.04.033.

26. Tuong W, Armstrong AW. Participant satisfaction with appearance-based versus health-based educational videos promoting sunscreen use: a randomized controlled trial. Dermatol Online J. 2015;21(2). http://www.ncbi.nlm.nih.gov/pubmed/25756492. Accessed March 29, 2019.

27. Tuong W, Armstrong AW. Effect of appearance-based education compared with health-based education on sunscreen use and knowledge: a randomized controlled trial. J Am Acad Dermatol. 2014;70(4):665–9. https://doi.org/10.1016/j.jaad.2013.12.007.

28. Tuong W, Wang AS, Armstrong AW. Effect of automated online counseling on clinical outcomes and quality of life among adolescents with acne vulgaris: a randomized clinical trial. JAMA Dermatol. 2015;151(9):970–5. https://doi.org/10.1001/jamadermatol.2015.0859.

29. Yentzer BA, Wood AA, Sagransky MJ, et al. An internet-based survey and improvement of acne treatment outcomes. Arch Dermatol. 2011;147(10):1223–4. https://doi.org/10.1001/archdermatol.2011.277.

30. Causa Research. https://www.causaresearch.com/. Accessed April 2, 2019.

31. Ferrándiz L, Morales-Conde M, Fernández-Orland A, et al. Teledermatology-driven topical therapy of actinic keratosis: a comparative study of clinical effectiveness and compliance. J Eur Acad Dermatol Venereol. 2018;32(12):2149–52. https://doi.org/10.1111/jdv.15085.

32. Wang SQ, Xu H, Dusza SW, Hu J, Stanfield J. Improving compliance of daily sunscreen application by changing accessibility. Photodermatol Photoimmunol Photomed. 2017;33(2):112–3. https://doi.org/10.1111/phpp.12292.

33. Sippel K, Seifert B, Hafner J. Donning devices (foot slips and frames) enable elderly people with severe chronic venous insufficiency to put on compression stockings. Eur J Vasc Endovasc Surg. 2015;49(2):221–9. https://doi.org/10.1016/j.ejvs.2014.11.005.

34. Lacour J-P, Paul C, Jazayeri S, et al. Secukinumab administration by autoinjector maintains reduction of plaque psoriasis severity over 52 weeks: results of the randomized controlled JUNCTURE trial. J Eur Acad Dermatol Venereol. 2017;31(5):847–56. https://doi.org/10.1111/jdv.14073.

35. Reich K, Zschocke I, Bachelez H, et al. A Topical Treatment Optimization Programme (TTOP) improves clinical outcome for calcipotriol/betamethasone gel in psoriasis: results of a 64-week multinational randomized phase IV study in 1790 patients (PSO-TOP). Br J Dermatol. 2017;177(1):197–205. https://doi.org/10.1111/bjd.15466.

36. Unrue EL, Cline A, Collins A, et al. A novel ultraviolet B home phototherapy system: efficacy, tolerability, adherence, and satisfaction. Dermatol Online J. 2019;25:2. http://www.ncbi.nlm.nih.gov/pubmed/30865405. Accessed April 1, 2019.

37. Höchsmann C, Infanger D, Klenk C, Königstein K, Walz SP, Schmidt-Trucksäss A. Effectiveness of a behavior change technique–based smartphone game to improve intrinsic motivation and physical activity adherence in patients with type 2 diabetes: randomized controlled trial. JMIR Serious Games. 2019;7(1):e11444. https://doi.org/10.2196/11444.

38. Lister C, West JH, Cannon B, Sax T, Brodegard D. Just a fad? Gamification in health and fitness apps. JMIR Serious Games. 2014;2(2):e9. https://doi.org/10.2196/games.3413.

39. Hoffmann C, Schweighardt A, Conn KM, et al. Enhanced adherence in patients using an automated home medication dispenser. J Healthc Qual. 2017;40(4):1. https://doi.org/10.1097/JHQ.0000000000000097.

40. Pillo Health. https://www.pillohealth.com/. Accessed April 2, 2019.

41. Schuman-Olivier Z, Borodovsky JT, Steinkamp J, et al. MySafeRx: a mobile technology platform integrating motivational coaching, adherence monitoring, and electronic pill dispensing for enhancing buprenorphine/naloxone adherence during opioid use disorder treatment: a pilot study. Addict Sci Clin Pract. 2018;13(1):21. https://doi.org/10.1186/s13722-018-0122-4.

42. Eichenfield LF, Krakowski AC. A novel patient support program to address isotretinoin adherence: proof-of-concept analysis. J Drugs Dermatol. 2015;14(4):375–9. http://www.ncbi.nlm.nih.gov/pubmed/25844611. Accessed April 2, 2019.

Index

© Springer Nature Switzerland AG 2020

S. R. Feldman et al. (eds.), *Treatment Adherence in Dermatology*, Updates in Clinical Dermatology,
https://doi.org/10.1007/978-3-030-27809-0